Differential Diagnoses

A VOLUME IN THE SERIES

The Culture and Politics of Health Care Work

edited by SUZANNE GORDON and SIOBAN NELSON

Differential Diagnoses

A COMPARATIVE HISTORY OF HEALTH CARE PROBLEMS AND SOLUTIONS IN THE UNITED STATES AND FRANCE

Paul V. Dutton

ILR Press *an imprint of*
Cornell University Press
Ithaca and London

First published 2007 by Cornell University Press
First printing, Cornell Paperbacks, 2008
Printed in the United States of America

Library of Congress Cataloging-in-Publication Data

Dutton, Paul V.
    Differential diagnoses : a comparative history of health
care problems and solutions in the United States and France /
Paul V. Dutton.
        p. cm.—(The culture and politics of health care work)
    Includes bibliographical references and index.
    ISBN 978-0-8014-4512-5 (cloth : alk. paper)
    ISBN 978-0-8014-7484-2 (pbk : alk. paper)
  1. Social medicine—United States—History—20th century.
2. Social medicine—France—History—20th century. 3. Medical
policy—United States—History—20th century. 4. Medical policy—
France—History—20th century. 5. Medical care—United States—
History—20th century. 6. Medical care—France—History—20th century.
7. Insurance, Health—United States—History—20th century. 8. Insurance,
Health—France—History—20th century. I. Title. II. Series.

    RA418.3.U6D88 2007
    362.1—dc22   2007010775

Cornell University Press strives to use environmentally
responsible suppliers and materials to the fullest extent
possible in the publishing of its books. Such materials include
vegetable-based, low-VOC inks and acid-free papers that are
recycled, totally chlorine-free, or partly composed of nonwood
fibers. For further information, visit our website at
www.cornellpress.cornell.edu.

Cloth printing   10 9 8 7 6 5 4 3 2 1
Paperback printing   10 9 8 7 6 5 4 3 2 1

Differential diagnosis: the distinguishing between two or more diseases with similar symptoms by systematically comparing their signs and symptoms.

Mosby's Pocket Dictionary of Medicine,
Nursing, and Allied Health

CONTENTS

PREFACE

My first book examined the twentieth-century development of France's social programs, including health care, retirement pensions, worker's compensation, and family welfare. As a result of years of research in France, my family and I have had considerable direct experience with French health care, from the neighborhood nurse who gives us our flu shots to the state-run well-child clinic that keeps our children healthy and vaccinated to the private-practice physicians who treat our occasional ailments. In the interest of full disclosure, the reader should know that our experiences have been overwhelmingly favorable. But so too has been our experience with U.S. health care. We are, after all, well insured and have the time and skills needed to negotiate the complexities of private U.S. medical coverage. Indeed, there is much to laud about health care and medical practitioners in both countries. This book, however, adopts a critical approach to health care through an international historical comparison. Only through an honest reckoning of the past will Americans and the French solve the truly daunting challenges that confront health care today.

Despite all my research and experiences on both sides of the Atlantic, I owe a tremendous debt to my colleagues who specialize in the welfare state of the United States and in the history of its health care. Without their penetrating work this book would not have been possible. I am equally indebted to health policy scholars of diverse disciplines whose work on present-day problems in France and the United States permitted me to bring this history into the contemporary period. Specialists from all these groups will, no doubt, find omissions in my analysis. This is only natural. I only ask that they bear in mind the breadth of the comparative project at hand. This request is also aimed at my fellow Europeanists. To behold a comparative picture, I have sometimes had to simplify my language and condense details so as to be understood by as broad an audience as possible on both sides of the Atlantic.

Many individuals gave gifts of time and expertise. Cecily Rometo served as my research assistant. Her analytical eye, incisive summaries, and attention to detail kept me on my toes and the project moving forward. Then there are those who carved out valuable time from their own research to provide professional advice. Timothy Smith and Bruno Valat read more chapter drafts than I can remember, but I will never forget their careful and insightful critiques. Michael Collier provided a discerning physician's view, which led to many improvements to the draft manuscript. Throughout it all, Suzanne Gordon of Cornell University Press made invaluable suggestions on behalf of a nonspecialist audience. Others provided precious encouragement, if only by suggesting yet another book to read or by reassuring me that what I was doing would eventually bear fruit. They include Herrick Chapman, Terry Clark, Leilah Danielson, Alexander Dracobly, Michel Dreyfus, Steve Early, Rachel Fuchs, Colin Gordon, Jeff Herf, Martha Hildreth, Romain Huret, Jennifer Klein, Cheryl Koos, Richard Kuisel, Jonah Levy, Sonya Michel, Allan Mitchell, Kimberly Morgan, Michael Osborne, Gail Radford, Jeremy Shapiro, Frank Sposito, Christopher Vaughan, and Neil Warrence. They contributed more to the project than they know.

This book could not have been completed without financial and institutional support. Grants from the United States Agency for Health Care Research and Quality and the National Endowment for the Humanities in 2001 and 2002 financed extended research sojourns in the United States and France. The Brookings Institution's Center on the United States and Europe did its share, underwriting the article from which I conceptualized much of the book. The Centre National de la Recherche Scientifique provided me with a forum for sharing my work and for making valuable contacts in Paris. The Woodrow Wilson International Center for Scholars gave me the perfect place to think and write, a refuge of reflection at 1300 Pennsylvania Avenue. I would like to thank the entire Wilson Center staff for their unstinting hospitality and support. Special mention must go to the Wilson Center's librarian Janet Spikes, without whose professional support I could not have included key statistical data. The Office of the Associate Provost for Research and Graduate Studies at Northern Arizona University also provided significant financial support. In addition, I would like to extend my appreciation to the chair of the history department at Northern Arizona University, Cynthia Kosso, for shielding my research from administrative and bureaucratic interruptions, a thankless but indispensable role for a university department chair. Finally, I owe the greatest thanks to my family. To Neil and Finley for understanding why their dad could not be there so many weekends. And to my best friend and wife, Shelby Reid, whose insights as a practitioner often provided a much-needed dose of firsthand knowledge to my historical analysis. Her confidence and commitment sustained me throughout the project.

Differential Diagnoses

1

COMMON IDEALS, DIVERGENT NATIONS

Healing is a matter of time, but it is sometimes a matter of opportunity.

HIPPOCRATES

Washington, D.C. I'm attending a good-bye party for a friend who is leaving her job at a local museum. A friendly group has gathered at a fashionable northwest restaurant for drinks and hors d'oeuvres. I find myself face to face with an art historian from the National Portrait Gallery. I get the standard question, "What do you do?" I tell the interrogator that I'm writing a book on U.S. and French health care. "Oh really," he responds. "Theirs is government imposed, isn't it?" Another scene. Flagstaff, Arizona. A Halloween party for kids, mostly of faculty from Northern Arizona University. I'm talking with a biologist. She asks about my research. I say it's on health care in France. I pause for the reaction, to which by now I've become accustomed. She replies, as if on cue, "You mean socialized medicine?" Back in Washington, at the Brookings Institution, a public policy research institute. It's intermission at a conference on transatlantic relations. I've just met a French businesswoman; she's curious about my work, so I recount the two scenes above. "Socialized medicine!" she exclaims in English, "That's the British!"

Americans often assume that all European health care systems are alike, something called "socialized medicine," under which the government, for good or ill, runs everything. Most do not understand that there are major differences among European countries in how they pay for and deliver medical care. More to the point, because European health care systems are dubbed—and dismissed as—"socialized medicine" Americans do not understand that they can learn much from how different health care systems address and resolve problems of cost, efficiency, and access. This is particularly important today as Americans consider how to cope with a health care crisis that often appears intractable.

By analyzing the historical development of the contemporary French and U.S. health care systems, I hope to advance this understanding, so that those concerned with health care policy in both countries—and ordinary citizens whose lives depend on the health care system—can avoid the pitfalls described by the historian Marc Bloch in his classic appeal on behalf of comparative history nearly a century ago. Bloch argued against the tendency to limit histories to one region or another. Historical research undoubtedly requires language expertise and in-depth knowledge of the society under scrutiny. Historians' specialization along regional and national lines has made possible enormous progress in understanding peoples and places on their own terms, free from any imperative to relate their past—or present—to some "other."

Yet with this practice of writing place-bound histories comes a certain danger. Authors quite naturally seek the causes and effects of the change they wish to describe within those boundaries. Much of the time they are justified in doing so. But in some cases, more general factors, which might be shared by more than one society or nation, go unnoticed. That is why Bloch advocated such a grand place for comparative history. Only through it, he believed, can we observe resemblances and differences across diverse lands and thereby perceive larger dimensions of the past that would otherwise remain unperceived, or worse, misperceived.[1]

In this book I present a comparative history of health care in the United States and France, from the early years of the twentieth century to the present day. I examine employers, labor unions, political groups, insurers, the state, and medical professionals to reveal their various influences on the French and U.S. health care systems and on the pursuit of health security by the citizenry of each nation. I consider not only what Americans have to learn from France but what the French have to learn from the U.S. example. Indeed, some of those on the U.S. side of the Atlantic who advocate a switch from the "french fry" to the "freedom fry" might be surprised to know how many values the two nations share and how much they are borrowing from one another. For example, the United States, quite by accident and with virtually no comprehensive planning or debate, is headed toward a public-private mix of health care financing that is far more French than most Americans realize. As a result, a better understanding of France's public-private health care system, its management, historical origins, and present challenges would be constructive in the U.S. search for health care solutions. The French, meanwhile, are busily adapting U.S. managed care techniques and hospital payment methods to their public and private health insurance. What more can these two countries learn and adapt (or adopt) from each other as they struggle with their respective health care crises?

What the French and U.S. health care systems share, as well as what divides them, is reflected in the various interpretations of their eighteenth-century revolutions. Both the American and French revolutionaries hailed the Enlightenment ideals of individual rights and popular sovereignty, leading to an inherent tension between personal liberty and social equality in the republics they formed.[2] This tension has been evident in virtually all health care reform initiatives since the First World War (1914–1918), which sought to compel citizens to participate in health insurance. Such debates have recurred on five occasions in the United States and twice in France. In each of these instances, a central question was whether individual liberty should be sacrificed for the sake of collective equality and the common good. In both countries, the debates exhibited nuanced arguments that sought to reconcile liberty and equality. Proponents argued that to compel a sacrifice on the part of the individual in the form of a small tax, would, in fact, free him or her from fear of medical indigence. The net outcome, they argued, was more liberty, not less. Meanwhile, opponents of compulsory health insurance consistently promoted voluntary measures, which made a powerful appeal to individual liberty, personal responsibility, and worker autonomy.

These questions remain at the heart of contemporary health care debates in both nations. How should one interpret the terms "liberty" and "equality" today? Does liberty require that health care be free from government intervention? Does equality entail equal access to medical care without regard for ability to pay? Or does it mean that insurers must take all comers? Should health care be linked to employment, as it is in both countries? How has this link constructed our views of the "deserving" and "less deserving" sick? How does one address the financial and professional concerns of vital health care actors, especially physicians? The tension between liberty and equality has been characterized in different ways over the course of the twentieth century: as personal responsibility versus social welfare, private enterprise versus communism, voluntarism versus compulsion, and individualism versus interdependent citizenship, to name a few. Just below the surface of all these designations lay fundamental tensions that were inescapable, given the founding ideals of both nations.

How History Helps Us Think about Contemporary
Health Care Challenges

Too often, health care studies, as informative as they are, offer only a snapshot, a single frame of what is inevitably a very long movie, whose directors, producers, and actors change the plot and the script in the course of the show. Relatively few policy studies deal in any depth with what are fundamentally historical causes and questions.

To begin with, U.S. and French health care was strikingly similar a hundred years ago. How and why did the two systems diverge so dramatically by century's end? And what about the similarities that remain, namely, the shared attachment to workplace health security; ideals of patient choice and private practitioners; and a common distrust of "socialized medicine"? This shared distrust has helped to conceal—certainly in the case of the United States—the fact that in all industrialized societies, health care has been socialized to a greater or lesser degree for a long time, and fortunately so. Few seriously ill patients or accident victims could pay the actual costs of the medical and hospital services they receive. Treatment for an auto accident can easily run into the tens of thousands of dollars. Depending on the model, a pacemaker, with installation costs, can come to over a hundred thousand dollars. Even fewer of us could afford the long-term nursing and valiant end-of-life care that has become common in the United States and Europe. In fact, 80 percent of health spending in the United States goes to care for just 20 percent of the population. It is roughly the same in France. Ten percent of its citizenry account for 60 percent of health care expenditures. If you are an average American or French reader, you will incur at least half of your lifelong medical expenses during your last six months of life. The burdensome cost of twenty-first-century health care simply has to be spread over large groups. What remains undecided is how best to do it.[3]

This is why, over the course of the twentieth century, countries developed two basic ways of socializing the cost of medical care to create health security for their citizenry. Great Britain possesses the archetypal *health service,* under which funding for most medical care facilities and the remuneration of doctors and other medical personnel flow more or less directly from the government treasury. In contrast, France and the United States rely heavily on *health insurance,* wherein medical facilities and health professionals are in both the public and private sectors, and their funding flows from public insurance funds and from private insurers.[4] France has large public health insurers, complemented by many private insurers. The United States presents a mirror image of this system. It relies heavily on large private insurers, which are supplemented by public health insurers such as Medicare. Throughout the twentieth century, France undertook successive reforms that encouraged physicians to remain in private practice, which doctors and patients alike believed was necessary to ensure ethical, quality care. Indeed, in France, discussion of a *service de santé* (a health service such as Britain's) elicits popular scorn in the same way that the term "socialized medicine" does in the United States. It is commonly viewed as antithetical to the nation's values.

In the United States, the term "socialized medicine" gained currency when opponents of President Harry Truman's national health insurance initiative in the late 1940s used it to characterize his program. As an epithet, it proved extremely effective because it bound together two emotionally charged concerns. First, it called to mind the United States' cold war with the Soviet Union and thereby tarred national health insurance as un-American and its backers as traitors. The president of the American Medical Association used to refer to proponents of national health insurance as having "a pinkish pigmentation," common parlance at the time for Communist sympathizers.[5] At the same time, "socialized medicine" invoked fear of impersonal, assembly-line medical care. Patients would not be able to choose their own doctor; medical personnel would owe allegiance not to the patient but to an anonymous and distant bureaucracy, which would require reams of paperwork and preauthorizations. Of course, as congressional testimony on the "Patient's Bill of Rights" aimed at health maintenance organizations (HMOs) in the 1990s demonstrated, impersonal treatment of patients can result from private medical bureaucracies just as well as from government ones. Yet that debate simply provides more evidence that Americans, like the French, possess strongly held beliefs about how patients should be treated and the limitations that reformers, whether public officials or private CEOs, face if they want to stem the rapidly rising cost of health care.

The United States and France share the distinction of possessing two of the world's most expensive health care systems. The U.S. system is far and away the more costly, gobbling up just over 15 percent of the gross domestic product (GDP), or $5,711, annually for every man, woman, and child in 2003. By 2014, the share of U.S. national income devoted to health care is expected to grow by nearly 25 percent, to 18.7 percent of the GDP. Meanwhile, the French have the fifth most costly health care system, spending almost 10.5 percent of their GDP, or $3,048, per capita in 2003. That share is also expected to rise, but not as quickly as in the United States. In both countries, health care price increases run at rates well above general inflation, driven by a host of factors, notably an unquenchable demand for increasingly effective (and expensive) diagnostic techniques and pharmaceuticals, and high salaries for expertly trained medical specialists. Both nations also have aging populations, which require on average far more hospital and medical services than younger groups.[6]

Though when all is said and done, the French get a lot more for a lot less money. In 2001, the World Health Organization (WHO) named French health care the best in the world. The United States ranked thirty-seventh in the same survey. For health policy experts in Paris and Washington, the WHO report did not come as a great surprise. France shone because of its universal insurance coverage, responsive health care providers, patient and practitioner freedoms, and the impressive health and longevity of its citizens. Although the United States scored at the top in some categories, such as provider responsiveness, its overall score suffered because of the astronomical cost of U.S. health care, its well-known problems for those without insurance (fully 15.9 percent of the population, or 46.6 million individuals in 2005), and the inequities in care depending on one's race, ethnicity, and socioeconomic status. One would have to return to the France of the 1960s to find the same levels of the uninsured and the shamefully poor access to medical care. Ninety-nine percent of the French population had obtained health insurance by 1980, either through public or private insurers, as a dependent of an insured person or through special funds for the unemployed. A 2000 law extended coverage to the remaining 1 percent that had somehow fallen through the cracks.[7] Public opinion in the United States and Europe reflects the high marks the WHO report gave to France.

A 2004 Harris poll of Europe's five largest nations found that the French are by far the most satisfied with their health care system (65 percent). By contrast, only 32 percent of Britons viewed their National Health Service in a positive light; the Germans panned their country's health care, with only 28 percent happy about its performance. When the same European respondents were asked which country's health care system they most admired, France again topped the list. Few Europeans in the survey felt positively about U.S. health care (10 percent), thereby agreeing with Americans themselves. A 2003 Kaiser Family Foundation poll found that 56 percent of Americans believed that their health care system needed major reform, while 30 percent expressed the view that it was beyond repair and should be completely rebuilt.[8]

While both nations face rapidly rising health care bills, price increases in the United States have been pushed further skyward by relatively high payroll expenses for nonmedical personnel, which includes underwriters, marketing specialists, insurance billers, and customer service agents. They

Table 1. American and French Demographic, Economic, and Health Indicators

Indicator	France	United States
Demography and Economics		
Total population (2004)	60,200,000	293,655,000
Population over 65 (2004)	16.3%	12.4%
GDP per capita (purchasing power parity) (2004)	$29,600	$39,700
GDP growth average (1994–2004)	2.3%	3.3%
Unemployment rate (2004)	10.1%	5.5%
Personal income tax of total receipts (2002)	17.3%	37.7%
Taxes on goods and services of total receipts (2002)	25.4%	17.6%
Average production worker's disposable income of gross pay (2002)	73.2%	75.7%
Health Care System		
Health care spending of GDP (2003)	10.4%	15.2%
Health care spending per capita (purchasing power parity) (2003)	$3,048	$5,711
Public portion of total health care spending (2003)	78.3%	44.6%
Practicing physicians per 1,000 residents (2004)	3.4	2.4
Physician consultations per capita (2003)	6.7	3.9
Acute care bed days per capita (2004)	1.0	0.7
Acute care beds per 1,000 residents	3.8	2.8
MRI scanner units per million residents (2004)	3.2	5.0
Health Status of Population		
Life expectancy at birth in years (2003)	79.4	77.5
Female life expectancy at 65 in years (2002)	21.4	19.5
Male life expectancy at 65 in years (2002)	17.1	16.6
Infant mortality per 1,000 live births (2003)	4.0	6.9
Tobacco consumption (percentage of population 15 years or older smoking daily) (2002)	26.0%	18.4%
Obese as percentage of population (body mass index > 30 kg m²) (2002)	9.4%	30.6%

Source: Compiled from *OECD in Figures 2005: Statistics on Member Countries* (Paris: OECD, 2005), 6–16, 38, and *OECD Health Data 2006* (Paris: OECD, 2006). Statistics for U.S. MRI units probably understate actual number since only the number of facilities with at least one unit is reported.

have become fixtures in the U.S. health care bureaucracy at health insurance companies, hospitals, clinics, and doctors' offices throughout the country. Meanwhile, analysts inside and outside France have observed that, far from conforming to stereotypes of a bloated government bureaucracy, French public health insurance, *Sécurité Sociale*, is probably understaffed.[9] Like Medicare and Medicaid in the United States, its administrative costs are well below those of private insurance companies (6 percent versus 13 percent).[10] The predominant role of *Sécurité Sociale* in French health care translates into a relatively high level of administrative efficiency compared with the United States. For example, instead of the labyrinth of deductibles, co-payments, and networks of medical care providers in the United States, a French patient presents a single microchip-enhanced *Sécurité Sociale* card at her physician's office. The card permits a physician online access to a comprehensive medical chart. It also implements an almost immediate electronic funds payment from *Sécurité Sociale* to the patient's bank account, reimbursing her for the appropriate portion of any fees associated with the doctor's visit. In addition to dealing with myriad health insurers, U.S. physicians have also faced large increases in their medical malpractice insurance premiums, as much as 30 percent in some states in 2004. French doctors have been spared these rising costs because the country's legal system is far more adverse to tort claims than its U.S. counterpart.

No matter what the reason for the rapid rise in health care expenditures, U.S. or French political leaders who talk of initiatives that threaten patient liberties or doctors' clinical freedoms do so at their peril. Like Americans, the French have never accepted and likely never will accept waiting lists for medical procedures, as Britons and Canadians do. "Rationing" is not a word on the lips of U.S. or French politicians, at least not among those who wish to enlist support for health care reform.[11] In 1995, when France's prime minister mentioned rationing care, if only to deny that his proposal included it, he suffered a devastating political defeat, as physicians rallied their patients to oppose him. That said, no matter what kind of system is used to allocate care, medical service providers inevitably respond, to a greater or lesser degree, to the financial incentives before them. Any financial incentive can bode ill or well for patient care and must be accompanied by ethical and legal safeguards. The fact remains, then, that in both the United States and France health care is rationed in myriad ways, based on ability to pay, statutory guidelines, administrative fiat, customary treatment regimens, and scientific practice norms, to name just the most common factors.[12] This being the case, it is clear that the aversion to "rationing" and "socialized medicine" in France and the United States is driven not by reason but by history, which it is critical to understand if we are to meet present-day challenges.

The Role of the State and the Workplace

It is difficult to imagine an institution more historically embedded in a nation's politics, economy, and culture than health care. For many social scientists, health care epitomizes a "path-dependent" creation. That is to say, at virtually every step of its development, specific conditions and events exerted formative influences that in turn induced others. As each critical historical juncture passed, its outcome influenced subsequent changes, making some results more likely than others.[13] The political scientist Margaret Levi has aptly compared such a process to climbing an old tree. The climber inevitably makes choices about which branch system to follow, and even though "it is possible to turn around or to clamber from one to another—and essential if the chosen branch dies—the branch on which a climber begins is the one she tends to follow."[14] This metaphor for how a nation's health care system evolves tells us that history matters, that singular historical moments can possess tremendous explanatory power, and that radical reversals may be hard to achieve.[15] But that does not mean that, because historical events on each side of the Atlantic are unique, the French and the Americans cannot learn how to solve their most nettlesome social problems from each other.

The French historian Alexis de Tocqueville understood this implicitly. He traveled widely in the United States during the 1830s, attempting to grasp the habits and institutions of the new nation in order to further his own understanding of France, especially its tribulations balancing liberty and equality. "In America," observed de Tocqueville, "free morals have made free political institutions; in France, it is for free political institutions to mould morals."[16] In this reflection, we see France's greater reliance on the republican state as an active agent in the quest for liberty and equality. After all, the French revolutionaries of 1789 faced a society far more rife with aristocratic privilege than the American colonies. In the revolution's most radical phase, under France's First Republic, its leaders tried and executed the king and queen, distributed the lands of the nobility and of the church to the peasantry, and banned slavery in France's colonies. These actions surely reflected the newly installed revolutionaries' willingness to use the state power that had once belonged to France's absolute monarchs, but they also showed a commitment to equality that American revolutionaries could only contemplate. Most notably, the founders of the United States refused to grant equality to nearly a million of their country-men and -women who had been forcibly brought to the States as slaves.[17]

De Tocqueville's remark also belies the influence of the eighteenth-century political philosopher Jean-Jacques Rousseau on French republi-canism. Next to inalienable individual rights, which are foundational to the republics of France and of the United States, Rousseau posited the exis-tence of a *general will*, a sort of infallible common good to which all citizens should (and must) submit.[18] But if the French republican state, even to the present day, can more easily intervene in the social and economic affairs of the nation, this does not mean there is no pluralism or protest in France's politics. On the contrary. As anyone who has witnessed French workers or students on strike will attest, those in the street can just as easily claim to possess the general will as those who occupy the government ministries. Indeed, France has experienced a fractious historical struggle over how to pay for and deliver health care, one that is just as contentious as that in the United States. By the same token, both countries have divided sharply over the state's power of compulsion. That explains why early in the twen-tieth century Americans and the French turned to nonprofit, independent associations that offered health security in the workplace.

In both nations, political leaders rightly surmised that highly centralized government-directed health care would be unpopular. Instead, they advo-cated a leading role for civil society organizations, considering them the best suited to reconcile liberty and equality in the pursuit of health. In France, these organizations were known as mutual aid societies, which long served as private health insurance clubs for stably employed men, usually through their workplace or professional association.

In 1930, French legislators empowered mutual societies to serve as insurance carriers under the country's first compulsory health insurance law. The lawmakers' decision was a compromise. They hoped to make compul-sory health insurance fit with France's longstanding tradition of voluntary, private approaches to health security. At about the same time, U.S. work-ers and employers were embracing Blue Cross, voluntary, nonprofit plans for group prepayment of hospital care, a model that was soon adapted for physician services under the name "Blue Shield." By the outbreak of the Second World War, employers and workers in both nations were sharing the risk of illness on an unprecedented scale by using nonprofit, nongov-ernment actors as intermediaries. In so doing, they preserved the traditional practices associated with private health insurance. Yet employment-based health security in both the United States and in France had unfortunate side effects where equality was concerned.

As some workers gained access to workplace health insurance, which they received in exchange for lower cash wages, they saw themselves (and were viewed by others) as responsible citizens who "deserved" any medical care they might need in the event of unexpected illness or accident. The "deserving" citizen was celebrated for his work and rewarded with health security. As defensible as this ethic may sound, its ugly underside was the belief that many citizens who, through no fault of their own, lacked access to workplace health insurance were "less deserving" of health security. Their only option was charity care, which did not come with the same guarantees of quality and patient choice that "deserving" citizens enjoyed. This development had a particularly negative impact on women and minorities, who were (and are) much more likely to be considered "less deserving."[19]

In both France and the United States, comprehensive health insurance— whether compulsory or voluntary— first became prevalent among industrial workers. Industry was a man's world where women were recognized only as adjuncts to the male worker's productive capacity. Most women worked at home and in nonmanufacturing jobs and could therefore gain insurance benefits only by virtue of their status as dependents. Employment-based health insurance thus served to reinforce decidedly unequal conceptions of gender and limited women's social mobility. Grouped with children as dependents of the male breadwinner, women were denied the dignity and liberties men enjoyed to pursue educational and employment opportunities.

In the United States, the industrial origins of health insurance affected agricultural workers in a similar manner and created disparities of health care access along racial and ethnic lines. By the late 1950s, most white unionized industrial workers in the northern and midwestern manufacturing centers had won generous health benefits at the collective bargaining table. Meanwhile, a disproportionate share of African American agricultural workers in the South, and of Latino farmworkers in the Southwest and California, lacked the economic and political power to obtain similar protections against illness and accidents.[20]

The notion of "deserving" and "less deserving" citizens persists in the United States and, despite the universality of Sécurité Sociale, even in France. In recent years, more and more middle- and upper-income French people have grown reliant on France's booming private supplemental insurance industry; these policies cover most of the difference between public insurance reimbursement and actual physician fees. Yet nearly 15 percent of the population lacks such coinsurance, meaning higher out-of-pockets costs for many who can ill afford it.[21] In fact, a recent study that controlled for socioeconomic, demographic, and health status factors found that French adults with supplemental insurance are 86 percent more likely to seek medical care than those without such coverage. This disparity nearly matches that found between the likelihood of insured and uninsured adult Americans seeking care, even though the financial burden of treatment for uninsured Americans is far greater than that for those who lack supplemental coverage in France.[22]

But nowhere is the distinction between "deserving" and "less deserving" citizens more apparent than in the U.S. health care program for the poor, Medicaid. Because Medicaid generally reimburses medical providers at lower rates than private insurers or Medicare, many clinics and physicians simply will not accept Medicaid patients. It appears to be a straightforward business decision, and physicians often justify it on those grounds. In a country with falling rates of private health coverage, however, Medicaid's inability to attract medical care providers exacerbates discrepancies in U.S. health care availability and quality. A 2005 study that measured quality and access to a set of core health services found that, a startling 85 percent of the time, poor people receive medical care of substantially lower quality than their higher-income compatriots. And that trend has worsened rather than improved in recent years.[23] Yet although low socioeconomic status has become the best predictor of an individual's quality of care, middle-income Americans still suffer serious consequences because of the nation's reliance on the workplace for health security.

Take the case of the San Diego physical therapist Amy D. Before September 2004 neither Amy nor her husband, Chris, would have viewed their family as vulnerable to health care insecurity. Amy, the daughter of a physician and sister of a surgeon, knew a great deal about health coverage through her family and her medical practice. She had been employed at the same clinic for six years; Chris worked for a small engineering firm through which they purchased comprehensive health insurance for themselves and their two children. In August 2004, however, Chris was laid off, leaving the family with two months to arrange new insurance. The following week, Amy was diagnosed with invasive breast cancer.

Because Chris's firm employed fewer than twenty employees (like 87 percent of all businesses, covering 19 percent of the U.S. labor force), the family could not take advantage of a federal law, known as COBRA, to buy continued group health coverage through Chris's workplace, even if he had been willing to pay both the employer and employee portions of the premium.[24] Meanwhile, Amy faced immediate surgeries and chemotherapy. She took a leave from her job on California state disability, which permitted her to purchase health insurance for herself through the clinic's Aetna group policy at six hundred dollars per month. Yet with Chris unemployed and Amy's disability stipend well below her usual income, the family could not afford the several hundred dollars more that would have been necessary to cover the entire family. Their home mortgage and mounting out-of-pocket coinsurance payments for Amy's treatment were just too high. Instead, they purchased catastrophic coverage for Chris and the children, which left Chris to seek care for his high blood pressure out of his own pocket. Yet this prudence only led to further health insecurity. When Chris landed a new job, his new employer's group policy excluded any coverage for illness related to his high blood pressure for one year, simply because he had wisely sought treatment for it.

Meanwhile, Amy's oncologist had placed her on Hercepton, an expensive (five thousand dollars per month) but highly effective treatment for some breast cancers. The regimen appeared to be working and Aetna was paying for most of it. But Chris's new employer group plan did not include Amy's oncologist in its provider network. Nor would the plan extend any dependent coverage at all if the employee's spouse could purchase coverage through her or his own workplace. Hence, because of Chris's new employment, which should have been cause for celebration, Amy had to quit a job she loved to gain affordable health coverage for the family. Even then, continuity-of-care imperatives for a life-threatening condition dictated that Amy remain with her original doctor, which she did, paying the 30 percent out-of-network coinsurance for Hercepton (fifteen hundred dollars a month) out of the family budget. Thankfully, Amy is a cancer survivor. Yet that status means that both she and Chris must forever weigh their employment decisions based on health insurance, not necessarily professional skill or salary.[25]

What happened to the D. family could not occur in France, because a series of reforms beginning in 1945 effectively severed the connection between an individual's employment status and health security. The sick, injured, or unemployed need not qualify for poverty assistance to enjoy public health insurance benefits, as they must in the United States. Indeed, unlike in the United States, the sicker you become in France, the greater your health care benefits. Inpatient hospital care for grave illnesses, for example, are covered 100 percent, while ambulatory care usually requires a steep coinsurance payment of 30 percent.

Yet France's past, when health security was dependent on employment, still exerts a powerful influence. Because of it, the French (like the Americans) continue to pay for their health insurance—and therefore much of their health care system—through paycheck deductions. French employers contribute 12.8 percent; workers pay .75 percent of wages and a 7.5 percent tax on wage and investment income.[26] Because of this reliance on payroll taxes, France is very different from Great Britain or Scandinavian countries such as Denmark, where diverse income and property taxes pay for 80 percent of the public health care system.[27] The French, even more than the Americans, possess a long enmity with income tax, and their government has relied on it only sparingly. In 2004, only 60 percent of all households were subject to income taxes, and even then the tax raises less than a fifth of government revenue, versus more than a third in the United States. France relies far more heavily on consumption taxes and payroll levies.[28]

Simple comparisons between U.S. and French health insurance payroll levies are difficult because of the wide array of U.S. medical insurance plans whose premiums vary by firm size and the "risk class" of the employees, a development whose origins I will explore in depth. Suffice it to say for now that U.S. health insurance is not priced as a percentage of wages, as in France, but in accordance with the health experience of the group or individual being insured. A large employer, such as the state of Arizona, which splits the cost of a family Blue Cross-Blue Shield preferred provider organization (PPO) plan with employees, paid over fifteen thousand dollars a year per enrollee in 2005. Hence, for a moderate-income earner (fifty thousand dollars annually), the cost of medical insurance relative to wages is significantly higher in the United States—30 percent, versus 21.3 percent—even for a large group purchaser like a state government. Similar Blue-Cross-Blue Shield coverage for small firms often costs much more. To be sure, some U.S. employers pay more than others toward their workers' coverage, but virtually all insist that rising health insurance premiums inevitably reduce cash wages. Thus, it was bad news for U.S. employers and workers when premiums for employer-based health coverage rose on average 7.7 percent in 2006, twice as fast as workers' wages (3.8 percent).[29]

In France, *Sécurité Sociale* health premiums flow into one of several public insurance funds—not the government treasury—and are jointly administered by employer and union representatives. Along with the government, *Sécurité Sociale* negotiates national medical fee schedules with the leading physician associations and other medical practitioner groups. These *conventions*, as they are called, form the basis of physicians' remuneration. Although close to a third of French physicians now charge fees above *convention* rates, their patients' reimbursement is tied to them.[30] Thus, as in the United States, where private insurers and Medicare use fee schedules to determine payments to physicians, French doctors' fees are ultimately constrained by insurers' willingness to pay.

Although a Frenchman or Frenchwoman's medical insurance no longer relies on a particular job, France's legacy of employment-based health security remains stubbornly evident in the joint administration of *Sécurité Sociale* by unions and employers. This arrangement has made health care reform extremely difficult, especially when the reform threatens the present reliance on paycheck deductions. Employers and labor leaders alike know that if health insurance premiums are "fiscalized," transferred away from payroll levies to a generalized income tax, their claims to control *Sécurité Sociale* governing boards would surely diminish, which could threaten their administrative prerogatives and generous worker benefits. This inertia in France's *Sécurité Sociale* is not unlike employers' and unions' addiction in the United States to the tax deductibility of health insurance premiums and policies, which are priced according to the policyholder's risk experience. These policies permit large employers and unions to purchase comprehensive health coverage at rates well below what small firms and individuals pay.

Workplace Health Security: An Artifact of the Twentieth Century

Workplace-related health security, whether through a direct link between employer and employee (as in the United States) or through public health insurance funds managed by labor and business leaders (as in France), are an artifact of the first half of the twentieth century. This artifact now hampers the resolution of health care crises in both nations. The downside of workplace-linked health insurance, which was embraced by workers and employers before and during the Second World War, now far outweighs its original civil society and associational benefits. Most obviously, there is a problem of equity. When one relies on wage levies to pay for health care, whole classes of income earners—those profiting from rents and investment dividends—make relatively small sacrifices yet still enjoy the most technologically advanced health care systems in the world. Even more damaging is the stultifying effect of workplace-related health security on employment freedom.

France has suffered from persistent high unemployment, nearly 10 percent, since the 1980s. At least some of this unemployment is caused by what economists call an "insider-outsider" problem.[31] "Insiders" are long-time employees with secure jobs; they enjoy good benefits, including *Sécurité Sociale,* as well as employer-provided supplemental health insurance. "Outsiders" are the unemployed or those in insecure, temporary positions. "Outsiders" would like a shot at an "insider" job but are stymied, not because they lack the skills but because employers face such high compulsory nonwage costs, for example, *Sécurité Sociale* payroll taxes. Employers hire only when they are absolutely certain that the new employee's additional productivity will translate into sufficiently higher and enduring firm revenues to justify the commitment. French employers also face far more cumbersome (and therefore costly) firing rules than their U.S. counterparts, rules that union leaders, who represent "insiders," are loathe to see weakened.[32] The end result, which is linked to France's payroll-financed health care, is that employers are reluctant to hire, leaving potentially productive workers in unemployment lines.

Well aware of this drag on employment, the French government in recent years has created a series of waivers whereby employers are excused from *Sécurité Sociale* charges, but only for a limited period. While this tactic has spurred hiring, somewhat driving unemployment down, it has also turned a stratum of France's workforce into temporary contract employees who are often let go when their employer's waiver expires. To be sure, because of *Sécurité Sociale* these workers enjoy far better health security during their temporary jobs and spells of unemployment than Americans in similar circumstances. Indeed, *Sécurité Sociale* maintains special health insurance funds for the unemployed and for those in unstable or seasonal work. Yet the link between employment and *Sécurité Sociale* remains an obstacle to more efficient labor markets and higher economic growth, which together constitute the most promising long-term solutions to France's high unemployment.

The relatively unregulated labor markets in the United States have helped it achieve higher levels of employment than France. That said, the United States appears to be developing its own version of the "insider-outsider" problem. As in the French case, this problem is closely tied to nonwage labor costs, but the U.S. version is even more directly caused by the health care system. A growing body of evidence shows that the U.S. economy suffers from "job lock" as a result of rising health care costs and health insurance underwriting practices.[33] Job lock occurs when a worker makes career decisions based on the imperative to maintain affordable medical insurance coverage or to avoid the exclusion of a preexisting condition for herself or for a family member.

Studies indicate that employer-provided health insurance reduces job mobility anywhere from 25 to 45 percent in the U.S. economy.[34] For economists, this is a frightening statistic, since the nation's economic health ultimately relies on an efficient match between workers' skills and their jobs. If a growing number of workers seek, first and foremost, not jobs where their skills pay them higher wages but jobs that provide them with good health insurance, then productivity and, eventually, economic growth and the U.S. standard of living will suffer. Most worrisome, this phenomenon is commonly observed at the cutting edge of economic innovation and entrepreneurship. Workers who might be most productive if they were to start their own firms choose not to do so because the self-employed and small firms face the highest health insurance costs. Needless to say, someone with a preexisting condition often cannot buy health insurance at any price to cover the malady and is therefore far more likely to remain in his or her current job, however unproductive.

Just as U.S. workers are limiting their own job choices in search of health security, employers too seek shelter from health care risks. This translates into employers' reluctance to take on full-time employees, instead favoring temporary and part-time workers, who are often ineligible for health benefits. Temporary workers' share of the labor market is growing far faster than the labor market as a whole.[35] Another response, which is not available to French employers, has been to screen workers for their potential health care costs to the company. In 2005, the nation's largest employer, Wal-Mart, promulgated plans to "dissuade unhealthy people from coming to work at Wal Mart."[36] Yet the far more common response, also an impossibility in France, is to reduce or drop health coverage altogether, or to transfer a greater share of cost increases to employees. The proportion of Americans under the age of sixty-five who received insurance from their employers (or a family member's employer) fell from 67.7 percent to 63.1 percent between 2000 and 2004. Employers who offered health coverage fell from 69 to 60 percent between 2000 and 2005.

Taken together, these developments explain much of the recent rise in the number of uninsured Americans. Although temporary workers and employees at small firms have been most affected, "insiders" in the United States—those who work in solidly unionized industries or for large firms—have also suffered from steep rises in their health insurance premiums. Between 2000 and 2005, premiums rose 73 percent, towering over the cumulative inflation rate (14 percent) and wage growth (15 percent).[37]

All this points to a tremendous irony. If current trends continue, Americans' historical attachment to employment-based private health insurance will lead inexorably to a publicly financed health care system. Workers who cannot find health security where it has traditionally been most available to them since the 1940s are already turning to Medicaid in unprecedented numbers, both during their working years and for nursing home care after they retire. Medicaid had more than 50 million beneficiaries in 2004, making it a larger program than Medicare. Meanwhile, those who earn too much to qualify for Medicaid but too little to afford private insurance join the ranks of the uninsured, a group that will grow to 56 million nonelderly adults by 2013, up from 45 million in 2003.[38] To be sure, the uninsured include young healthy adults who forgo coverage of their own volition. Yet whether by choice or not, when serious illness or accident strikes, the uninsured inevitably rely on some level of care at public expense, even as they themselves face financial ruin. Add to this the nearly $600 billion cost of the new Medicare prescription drug benefit and total U.S. national health expenditures will shift from being primarily private to being mostly public by 2014.[39] What is more, these calculations do not even include lost government revenue (a form of public subsidy) as a result of employers' and employees' health insurance tax deductions, valued at $188 billion in 2004, a number that has been growing at a 9.2 percent annual rate since 1998.[40]

The legacy of workplace-linked health security must be recognized for what it is—a twentieth-century solution that is failing to solve twenty-first-century health security problems. Because of its extraordinary cost, U.S. health care, like the French, has now passed from being primarily a private affair to a public-private endeavor. With this shift, the burdensome link between employment and health security has become all the more evident.

Liberty, Equality, and Medicine

Much of this book concerns the response of physicians to various health care challenges. During the twentieth century and into the present, French and U.S. physicians have had a common political ideology, espousing the medical profession's sovereignty over health care. Doctors' struggle to defend their clinical freedoms and medical decision making has long been aided by a shared U.S. and French attachment to private practice, under which doctors and other medical care providers are paid for each individual service. In its purest form, fee-for-service medicine—*paiement à l'acte* in French— permits patients to choose their own doctors and physicians to set their own fees. Equally important, proponents of fee-for-service medicine historically protected the sanctity of the doctor-patient relationship with almost religious fervor, especially against any encroachment by the state.

Doctors' battles against government plans for compulsory health insurance were enormously important in shaping the health care systems of both nations. French physicians agreed to cooperate with compulsory health insurance plans for industrial workers only in 1930, when they obtained valuable guarantees regarding their right to set fees, exercise clinical freedoms, and allow a patient to choose the practitioner. Likewise, U.S. physicians, though fiercely opposed to Medicare in the early 1960s, ultimately obtained similar assurances that protected their clinical freedoms vis-à-vis the state. What is often overlooked, however, is that private insurers—not the state—have historically posed the greater threat to physicians' sovereignty over medical decision making and to a patient's choice of health care provider.

French mutual aid societies served as insurance carriers for compulsory health insurance in the 1930s. Much as U.S. managed care corporations would do in the 1980s and 1990s, mutual societies threw vast resources into building clinics and surgery centers, then staffed them with doctors whom they compensated through a combination of capitation and salary.[41] Patients who patronized these facilities enjoyed lower out-of-pocket costs, but their choice of physician was limited, and financial incentives that might have conflicted with their best interests were ever-present. By providing medical services in much the same way that managed care does today, mutual societies directly violated legal protections of French physicians' fee-for-service practice, leading to successful legislative, legal, and professional action against the offending societies and complicit doctors.

At about the same time, the American Medical Association (AMA) launched professional and legal attacks against group medical practices, such as Kaiser Health Plans, which accepted prepayment for services and restricted a patient's choice to doctors in the plan. In these battles, the AMA usually prevailed. But they lost the war. Lacking the legal protections of private-practice medicine that French doctors gained in successive compromises on national health insurance, U.S. physicians were overwhelmed in the 1990s by a coalition of employers and insurers who sought lower prices through managed care. A new generation of U.S. physicians was soon signing up with managed care corporations, which now monitor doctors' treatment regimens, doling out incentives and punishments, in ways that would have horrified their elders.

Because of the continued upward spiral of health care costs in France, physicians there are under similar, if less heavy-handed, pressure to abide by clinical practice norms. Indeed, if U.S. health care is becoming more French in its reliance on public funds, France's *Sécurité Sociale* is behaving more and more like a U.S. managed care corporation. Recent reforms have made *Sécurité Sociale* increasingly assertive in its quest to curb hospital stays, pare physicians' use of expensive diagnostic technologies, and mold their habits for prescribing drugs. In fact, the health policy scholar Victor Rodwin has labeled France's ongoing reforms "the birth of state-led managed care." With the introduction of computerized medical records, medical practice guidelines, and gatekeeping primary care physicians, *Sécurité Sociale* hopes to take what it deems the best from U.S. managed care but leave its more unpopular initiatives behind.[42] The strategy has an appeal. Because nearly 99 percent of France's ambulatory care doctors contract with *Sécurité Sociale,* French patients will never face the maze of provider networks and exclusionary underwriting practices that hamper quality, access, and continuity of care in the United States.

Nevertheless, though France's relatively centralized public insurance system appears a promising candidate for managed care techniques, there is a powerful cultural counterforce rooted in the nation's historical embrace of individualism. Not unfamiliar to Americans, it absolutely rejects the notion that any individual's medical treatment should be weighed against a theoretical allocation of scarce resources for the common good. Of course, such financial cost-benefit analyses lie at the heart of managed care's resource allocation efficiencies and cost control. The tremendous value placed on the individual, combined with physicians' sovereignty over medical decision making, means that French health care reforms that rely on managed care techniques will continue to face difficult if not insurmountable obstacles.[43] What is clear is that in both nations, physicians' diagnostic, prescriptive, and therapeutic liberties remain at odds with efforts to rationalize health care, control its costs, and spread its benefits.

Medical Practice Then and Now

As a starting point, we should recognize that at the beginning of the twentieth century, medicine in France and the United States closely resembled each other in both practice and ideals. Medical science had only recently begun to make good on its ambitious promises. In France, the discoveries of Louis Pasteur established the prestige of scientific medicine, setting it apart from popular and folk medicine for the treatment of infection and the promotion of public health. The German Robert Koch identified the tubercle bacillus, thereby demonstrating the power of medical science to isolate the cause of the era's most feared killer, tuberculosis. Also extremely important were improvements in anesthesia, which, by relieving pain, permitted surgeons—then a far less respected branch of practitioners than physicians—to perform what had been impossible procedures on the body's major organs.

Yet the empirical and theoretical case for scientific medicine took decades to advance. The late 1800s were not the late 1900s when discoveries and improved techniques could be quickly shared across the globe. Well into the twentieth century, folkways and patent medicines of dubious value held sway. What mattered most to people, then as now, were results. And since medical science could often do little better than the traditional treatments, and often simply waited for the malady to run its course, the public had nowhere near the respect for doctors that they do today. Physicians' socioeconomic status has always closely reflected the effectiveness of the medical science of their day; this relationship helps us understand physicians' response to health care change.

Had we been able to eavesdrop on a conversation between two typical general practice doctors, one American and one French, posted to the western front during the First World War, in 1917, their conversation would have attested to ideological and practical kinship. Reminiscing about their lives back home, the physicians would have found they had both been raised in petty bourgeois families and had been drawn to medicine in hopes of earning a respectable but not lavish income. Their solo medical practices relied on tiresome travel between rural and working-class households struck by illness. Both doctors would have bemoaned miserly contracts, which, out of financial necessity, they had signed with mutual aid societies or fraternal lodges—contracts that bound them to treat the group's entire membership for a low fixed price. The two practitioners would have been equally upset with industrialists who resisted paying them on a fee-for-service basis, wanting instead to make them mere employees in their growing enterprises. Their loudest exhortations, however, would have been reserved for their respective governments: both would have sworn to fight any further government meddling in medical care, now that workers' compensation laws had been fully implemented in France and American state governments were approving them at a lively pace.[44]

This Franco-American camaraderie would have stood in stark contrast to the circumstances and ideals of doctors on the other side of the barbwire or to those of a British physician who happened to be standing nearby. Germany had created Europe's first compulsory health insurance for about 4 million industrial workers in 1883, a move that drastically affected the relationship between doctors and their patients, and between doctors and the government. Indeed, if our U.S. and French doctors had been able to share editorials from their medical journals, they would have seen that in both nations medical leaders defined virtually all that was good and noble about medicine by contrasting it with anything and everything German. Likewise, British doctors had flocked to Britain's National Insurance Act, passed in 1911, which, though less constraining than German illness insurance, nonetheless put the country squarely on the side of government-directed health care.

Today, a comparable conversation between two typical primary care physicians in private practice—great-granddaughters, let us say, of our World War One comrades—would also attest to sociological and practical kinship. A typical physician in both nations is nearly as likely to be a woman as a man, and she is very likely to hail from a professional, upper-middle-class family—a daughter of a doctor or lawyer, not a baker. As important as these commonalities may be, the great-granddaughters would find many more differences in their practices than had their great-grandfathers. Virtually all the French physician's patients would be eligible for public health insurance, *Sécurité Sociale*, a circumstance shared by the U.S. doctor only if she restricted her care to Medicare and Medicaid patients, not a common practice. The U.S. doctor's income would be much higher, just over five times the average U.S. wage, while the French doctor would earn only about twice the average earnings of her compatriots. As a primary care practitioner, however, the French doctor would·have many more colleagues, about half of all doctors in France, and a relatively easy time flying solo in her own office. Primary care physicians constitute only about a third of U.S. doctors and, because of the almost overarching need to hire non-medical personnel to handle the cumbersome and various insurance billing procedures, solo medical practices are now far less common in the United States. Despite differences in their offices, both physicians would surely agree that the radically higher incomes of specialists in both countries were out of proportion to their extra training. Primary care physicians work just as hard, they would insist, and entrance to medical school is fiercely competitive in France and in the United States, regardless of whether one plans to pursue a specialty. Finally, for all her envy of her U.S. colleague's higher income, the French doctor could take comfort that she paid only nominal malpractice insurance premiums and had never borrowed to pay medical school tuition. Like all French universities, medical schools are tuition free. If the U.S. practitioner recounted her travails with insurers and her occasional practice of "defensive medicine" to guard herself against lawsuits, the French physician might conclude that doctoring in France may be less remunerative, but it is considerably more hassle-free.[45]

The patients these physicians admitted to hospitals would also be very different from their early-twentieth-century predecessors. At that time, aside from facilities for veterans, which have illustrious histories in both nations, hospitals were local institutions. Most were owned and operated by municipalities, religious groups, or nonprofit organizations whose mission included community service, for example, universities, which built teaching hospitals for their medical students. Publicly traded, for-profit hospital chains were unknown.[46]

Today, France's hospital sector is dominated by community and university hospital medical centers. Yet, as with ambulatory care, where private insurers round out public coverage, private hospitals (both for profit and nonprofit) offer care that complements inpatient services in the public sector. In fact, France possesses the largest private hospital sector in Europe, accounting for 36 percent of all beds for acute cases, a public-private mix that has not changed in the last fifteen years. Generally, the patients with the most serious and complex cases end up in public hospitals, with private hospitals specializing in more routine obstetrics, elective and cardiac surgery, psychiatric care, and radiation therapy. Ultimately, however, the choice of hospital is up to the patient, his or her *Sécurité Sociale* coverage being the same in both the private and public sectors.[47]

Public community hospitals now account for only a quarter of hospitals in the United States. Moreover, in contrast to its French counterpart, the U.S. hospital sector has witnessed a vast transformation in its public-private mix in recent decades. Between 1985 and 1995, the number of public hospitals declined by 14 percent. Of these, nearly two-thirds converted to private ownership or management, while the remainder closed their doors entirely. Hence, once again, as in the case of public versus private health insurance, the United States and France present mirror images of each other in their emphasis on public versus private ownership or control.

The phenomenon of U.S. hospital closures provides a poignant example of how and why comparative historical approaches to health care are vitally important. U.S. observers generally attribute the closures to a 1980s switch from cost-plus reimbursement (under which hospitals charged insurers their actual costs plus a margin) to a case-based system (whereby hospitals are paid according to the patient's diagnosis). The resulting incentives translated into shorter hospital stays and therefore a decline in the total number of beds, since longer patient stays cost the hospital more without increasing its revenues.[48] Certainly there is something to this explanation. Yet France also adopted case-based hospital reimbursement in the 1980s. Indeed, it was the first country outside the United States to do so. But France has maintained its relatively high ratio of beds per capita—3.8 per thousand compared with 2.8 per thousand in the United States. And France continues to do so at lower costs. The answer to this paradox is best apprehended through a historical approach, wherein health care is viewed not just in technical terms but also as a nexus of culture, politics, and economics.

The Pitfalls of Language

A history of health care, especially a comparative one, faces several pitfalls. Language is perhaps the most treacherous. One cannot blithely assume that words possess a constant meaning over time and in different countries.[49] To begin with, the same political term may have very different meanings on either side of the Atlantic, both historically and in contemporary usage. *Liberalism* in France denotes political beliefs that most would identify with fiscal conservatives or libertarians in the United States: advocacy of markets, deregulation, private enterprise, and balanced government budgets. Indeed, a private-practice physician who insists on billing and clinical freedoms in France is known as a "liberal doctor" (*un médecin libéral*); and the burgeoning private-practice medical sector is known collectively as "liberal medicine" (*la médecine libérale*). For the sake of clarity in both interpretation and translation, I use functional terms in the pages that follow—for example, *private-practice*—that correspond with their practical signification in time and place.

Another lexical difficulty in comparing U.S. and French institutions concerns *the state*. The distinction between the United States' federal and state governments is readily apparent. The term "French state" (*l'Etat français*), however, often capitalized in French documents, includes a civil service whose power relative to the elected government is greater than its U.S. counterpart. To be sure, the federal bureaucracy is no pushover when a new U.S. president wishes to implement substantial change, nor can any governor in the country assume that her state bureaucracy will cooperate fully when directed to execute reform.

Yet in France's more unified political structure, bureaucrats, especially high officials, who usually devote their careers to public service, enjoy an autonomy and public trust not present in the United States. The founding director of *Sécurité Sociale*, Pierre Laroque, is a preeminent example. Very few Americans could name the first director of a comparably popular domestic program, such as Social Security or Medicare. By contrast, in France, it is Laroque, not the prime minister who held the reins of government in 1945, who is widely known and celebrated as "the father" of *Sécurité Sociale*. Yet Laroque was never elected to any office. Indeed, in high state officials, as much as anywhere else in Paris, resides Rousseau's general will, that is, a public perception of the common good. Thus, more so than in the United States, when private interests look to the state to arbitrate a conflict, implement reform, or simply guarantee their rights, they are appealing as much to an elite administrative corps as to elected political leaders.[50]

Next, we must address several terms related to health. A *health care system* today comprises the totality of activities, actors, and institutions devoted to the financing of efforts to prevent, treat, and cure illness or injury. By that definition, the U.S. and French health care systems touch almost every aspect of our societies—from employers to governments to schools to places of worship, not to mention health care providers, insurers, and patients. Yet *health care system* is certainly not a term that would have been understood by someone in 1900. At that time, the broadest comparable concept would have been *public health*, which encompassed the concepts of hygiene, living conditions, and medical facilities that were largely devoted to charity care.[51]

In the same way, a *hospital* of 1900 had little in common with today's gleaming medical complexes, staffed as they are by highly trained specialists, equipped with sophisticated diagnostic tools, and filled with effective pharmaceuticals. Hospitals at the turn of the twentieth century were social prisons, hostels for the helplessly destitute, the chronically ill, the tubercular, and the insane. For its residents, the hospital may have been better than the street, but it was not a place where one went to get well. The transformation of hospitals into sought-after centers of curative care did not gain speed until between the world wars.

Today, Americans fret about *health security*. The term evokes the specter of rising insurance premiums and the loss of insurance coverage; bankruptcy caused by medical debts; and tragic cases of medical indigence—the complete loss of financial well-being resulting not from a debilitating illness or accident but from the expenses associated with it. Indeed, 54.5 percent of Americans who filed bankruptcy in 2001 cited medical expenses as a primary cause.[52] *Health security* in 1900—to the extent that such a concept was even conceivable—had little to do with medical bills. If you were a stably employed man, you might be able to obtain *illness insurance*; its main purpose, however, was not to pay doctors' bills but to replace lost earnings if you were unable to work. Wage loss because of sickness or injury was one of the leading causes of pauperization in the nineteenth century, and usually amounted to far more than the cost of a patient's medical treatment. Nineteenth-century reformers thus viewed illness insurance as an antipoverty measure with only indirect implications for medicine and health care.

Even the definition of *health* has changed dramatically over the twentieth century. Early in the century, *health* commonly meant the absence of physical disease or injury. Those who could walk, talk, and work were deemed healthy. By 1970, *health* had become as much a state of mind as a definition of bodily ability. Not only had mental fitness been added to the definition of health; rapid advances in medicine enabled undreamt-of improvements in the quality of life. Through a new awareness of diet and exercise, health began to be perceived as a process as well as a condition. A mutually reinforcing dynamic took hold, creating an unquenchable demand for health care services. Breakthroughs in medicine and technology stoked the demand for medical care, which in turn pushed the standard of "good health" constantly higher. Today, the vast resources devoted to easing the discomforts of aging, to restoring everything from skin color to penile function, and the heroic efforts to extend life itself, however miserable or unconscious that life might be, make the pursuit of *health* look like a quest for immortality. In an important sense, then, this book is as much about how the Americans and the French, attached as we are to the ideals of liberty and equality, have pursued changing notions of *health* as it is about the actors and institutions that seek to protect and maintain it.

A Road Map

In this book, I trace the development of medical care and health insurance beginning at the time of the First World War (1914–1918). The Great War, as it was then known, was a watershed in both nations. It marked the United States' first large-scale debate over whether health insurance should become compulsory or remain voluntary. Through its victory in the war, France regained territories in Alsace-Lorraine, which it had lost to Germany in the Franco-Prussian War of 1870. This presented a conundrum for French leaders. France's new citizens in Alsace-Lorraine had grown fond of Germany's public health insurance. Thanks in large part to circumstances in Alsace-Lorraine, by 1930 French reformers had won their battle for compulsory health insurance, while their U.S. counterparts had lost theirs. Their victory put France on a path toward health security that privileged public coverage and used private measures as a supplement, a mirror image of the course the United States would take.

Yet these differing choices between public compulsion and private voluntarism are only part of the story. The debates in France and the United States over health insurance energized doctors on both sides of the Atlantic, prompting expansive claims of professional sovereignty from the fledgling U.S. and French medical associations. Through these debates, but in very different ways, doctors in both nations won professional autonomy in the form of fee-for-service private-practice medicine, an institution that would become a paradigm in France and the United States for much of the rest of the century.

In subsequent chapters, I turn to the indispensable role of civil society groups in spreading health coverage during the 1930s and 1940s, especially mutual aid societies in France and Blue Cross in the United States. As nonprofit organizations with public service missions, both enjoyed wide popularity because of their valued role as intermediaries between employers, the market, and the state. That said, doctors also treated both organizations with great suspicion and occasional hostility. Yet U.S. medical leaders reserved even greater animosity for President Franklin Roosevelt's New Deal. Chapter 3 analyzes why health coverage was not included in the 1935 Social Security Act, pointing to the opposition of southern legislators, employers, and physicians. The failure to enact health insurance alongside the New Deal's compulsory pension program (Social Security) was perhaps the most important thing that did not happen in the history of U.S. health care. For it created a vacuum in which Blue Cross, and later, Blue Shield could thrive. Their success was quickly followed by commercial insurers, whose increasingly refined abilities to assess risk induced a disposition toward exclusion in U.S. health insurance practices that has proved difficult to reverse.

Chapter 4 takes up the Second World War, drawing structural parallels and distinctions between the health care initiatives associated with the New Deal in the United States and those of France's wartime regime based in the spa town of Vichy. Both governments espoused maternal and rural ideals, offering generous medical care programs to expectant mothers and rural inhabitants hardest hit by the Depression. In both cases, however, these ideals were constructed on highly gendered and exclusionary bases. I also examine the corporatist arrangements that governed management-labor relations and how they influenced the development of employment-based health coverage in both nations during and after the war.

The liberation of France from Nazi occupation in 1944 heralded the creation of *Sécurité Sociale,* whose leaders made far-reaching promises of greatly expanded health coverage based on the principle of national solidarity. Yet the nature and price of that coverage remained difficult to manage. Chapter 5 analyzes the struggles of French and U.S. labor unions to maintain influence over their members' health care benefits after the war. The emergent definition of health as a state of complete physical and mental well-being boosted the demand for health care services. Increased demand joined with more effective and expensive medical techniques to bring about rapid rises in health care costs. In France, labor leaders dominated the nation's *Sécurité Sociale* boards, but they still could not prevail over hospitals or physicians to hold down fees, thereby avoiding sharp hikes in workers' out-of-pocket expenses. Meanwhile, U.S. union leaders tried but failed to gain influence on Blue Cross boards and suffered Blue Shield's rebuke when they pursued measures that would have lowered patients' out-of-pocket expenses. Thus union leaders in both countries watched helplessly as doctors, under the banner of professional liberty, adopted what came to be known as "usual, customary, and reasonable" fees.

The French and U.S. governments' responses to the health care inflation of the 1950s could not have been more different. Their contrasting choices are the focus of chapter 6. In 1960, President Charles de Gaulle forcefully trimmed doctors' billing freedom by insisting that doctors abide by negotiated fee schedules. Most U.S. political leaders, meanwhile, continued to equate direct state intervention in health care with Communism and the destruction of the American way of life. They favored the tax deductibility of group insurance premiums, a powerful if indirect measure that bolstered employers' role in the provision of health security. In pursuit of further savings, U.S. unions and employers embraced experience-rated insurance policies to hold down premium increases, a move that gradually left retirees as well as workers and their dependents from poor and unorganized sectors of the economy permanently outside employment-based coverage. The move on the part of the United States to experience-rated insurance and away from community rating further committed the country to private, employer-based, voluntary insurance for the gainfully employed and made compulsory health coverage for retirees (Medicare) and state-financed care for the poor (Medicaid) virtually inevitable. It had simply become too risky to insure the elderly and the poor without forceful state action.

Chapters 7 and 8 address the decades after 1970, when health care cost control moved definitively to the fore in both nations. If U.S. political leaders had earlier spurned French-style medical fee schedules when creating Medicare, they now embraced an innovative hospital fee schedule known as Diagnosis Related Groups. Not surprisingly, France was the first nation to test and deploy DRGs outside the United States. But Prime Minister Raymond Barre also believed that the solution to health care inflation lay in taking advantage of market forces in order to dampen health care demand and spur competition between providers. In an attempt to do so, France permitted physicians the freedom to raise fees well above levels that had been negotiated between *Sécurité Sociale* and doctors' groups. Within a few years, however, government and medical leaders alike judged the reform dangerous to health care access. Yet it has proved difficult to reverse.

Back in the United States, physicians were losing billing freedoms, not gaining them. A 1973 federal law that encouraged the creation of health maintenance organizations had finally taken hold, with corrosive effects on doctors' sovereignty over medical decision making. In contrast to the New Deal and Great Society eras, the 1990s saw employers drown out doctors' protests with their howls about skyrocketing premiums. Indeed, for a while, managed care succeeded in slowing health care inflation, earning a central role in President Bill Clinton's ill-fated 1994 reform proposal. But medical inflation soon reasserted itself, now combined with an ever-increasing number of uninsured Americans.

French political and medical leaders closely watched Clinton's health care reform efforts. In 1995, Prime Minister Alain Juppé launched his own plan, attempting to avoid Clinton's mistakes, but to no avail. Chapter 8 analyzes the Clinton and Juppé failures, focusing on the discord that proposals for universal health insurance produce—whether among covered Americans who fear that reform will threaten their employer-based insurance (like those portrayed in the "Harry and Louise" television spots against the Clinton plan) or among French workers who fear that their generous benefits will be trimmed as part of unproven measures for health care savings. This theme is carried forward in the concluding chapters, where I trace the historical provenance of the most recent reforms, including France's attainment of universal coverage in 2000, the Medicare Modernization Act of 2003, health savings accounts, and ongoing efforts by France's *Sécurité Sociale* to implement managed care techniques such as gatekeeping physicians and practice norms. Throughout, liberty and equality, public versus private, and individualism versus interdependent citizenship provide the philosophical frameworks for the analysis.

2

HEALTH INSURANCE AND THE RISE OF PRIVATE-PRACTICE MEDICINE, 1915–1930

A doctor is at no one's service, earning no wages; he makes a living only from his clientele who entrust him with their care. His sole masters are and must be his conscience and his professional honor…his sole purpose the interest of his patients; he is a completely independent man!

FANTON D'ANDON, President of the Syndicat des Médecins de la Seine, 1925

The First World War (1914–1918) marks the end of what historians call "the long nineteenth century." The war brought about such rapid social, political, and economic change that the first president of the United States elected after the conflict, Warren Harding, vainly coined a new word, "normalcy" to promise Americans a return to a bygone era. As the bloody site of most of the fighting, France also yearned for a return to what many now termed *la belle époque* of the turn of the century. So it is altogether fitting that the evolution of health care during the early twentieth century should reflect both the realities of a newly transformed world and an idealized conception of the past.

In France and the United States, the early twentieth century witnessed a renewed prominence of fee-for-service private-practice medicine, a development that would shape health care in both nations for much of the century. The attributes of private practice—patient choice of doctor, direct payment of medical fees for each service rendered, the physician's freedom to diagnose and prescribe, and the confidentiality of doctor-patient relations—became the subject of intense political battles elsewhere, but nowhere was its victory more complete than in France and the United States.

As familiar as private medicine appears to us today, it was far from predominant in the early twentieth century. For many physicians, a fee-for-service private practice was only a dream, a vision of physician autonomy in which fraternal orders and company bosses played no role. In this ideal, the doctor's clinical gaze extended beyond the patient to the patient's home, where so much of the medicine of the day was practiced.[1] Having seen the house and knowing the family, he set his fees accordingly, perhaps even waiving them altogether. If he submitted a bill, he expected payment directly from the patient, not some anonymous third party. The opponents of compulsory health insurance in both nations were especially fired by their aspirations for private-practice fee-for-service medicine and the professional sovereignty it entailed.

The special legitimacy of liberty in the United States and France granted them a cultural authenticity that ultimately proved irresistible. In the debate over compulsory health insurance, a patient's free choice of physician was posited as a natural right. A doctor's clinical freedom and medical confidentiality emerged as inalienable from the practice of medicine. Direct payment of unregulated fees was cast as fundamental to physicians' liberty. In short, according to its backers, the principles of private practice were truths deemed self-evident. And anyone who dared question them could not be considered entirely "American" or "French." This is not to say that advocates of other forms of medical practice, which may have better matched emergent social conditions of the early twentieth century, lacked an attractive rhetoric of their own. They appealed to the value of equality, "fair play," health security for all workers, and the good of the nation. Liberty versus equality—these were the themes on which the first battles over compulsory health insurance were fought in both nations. And fought they were. Unlike any other in the history of health care, the debate divided workers, employers, insurers, government officials, and especially physicians. It raised fundamental questions about health security, questions that the Americans and the French still grapple with today. What rights can workers as patients claim? What powers should employers as payers rightfully retain? And what role must government play?

France's debate differed greatly from its U.S. version, most notably in its outcome. French leaders reached a compromise that incorporated the country's highly regarded insurers, known as mutual aid societies, into a system of compulsory health insurance. Yet at least as important as this contrast is a striking similarity. In both countries the debate over health insurance resulted in the reinforcement of fee-for-service private medicine as the most legitimate form of medical practice, both legally and ethically. Unprecedented in the history of health care, this development is still very much with us. All proposed changes to health care, whether in the public or the private sector, have been and are scrutinized for their congruence with its principles. Many reforms over the course of the twentieth century have succeeded or failed based on whether they passed muster.

In light of this doctrinal uniformity, which had become entrenched in both countries by 1930, it is instructive to note that participants in this earliest debate over compulsory health insurance—from employers to trade unionists, from doctors to insurers—were riven by internecine struggles. The long-forgotten views of those who lost these internal battles tell us much about the virtues and frailties of health care in France and the United States today. Let us begin with the reformers' motivations in each nation and the various models of health security that vied for their attention.

A Progressive Age

The nature of health care is inextricable from modernity. By this I mean not merely the stupendous technological advancements and specialization that mark modern medical care at present but also the larger social and economic transformation brought about by industrialization and urbanization. In 1860, less than a fifth of Americans lived in cities; by 1910 nearly half did. During the same fifty years, nonagricultural workers jumped from 42 percent to nearly 70 percent of the labor force. France exhibited a similar acceleration in the growth of cities and industrial employment. Early-twentieth-century health care reform movements in both countries were closely tied to more general efforts to safeguard living standards in the face of large-scale industrial capitalism. Progressives, as they were loosely called in the United States, and *solidaristes*, a still-revered political label in France, were the principal architects of many of these initiatives.

American Progressives are perhaps best known for their successful early legislative initiatives to protect the health and safety of workers and consumers. The Pure Food and Drug Act, the Meat Inspection Act, workplace safety and child labor laws, and worker's compensation are all examples of Progressive reforms. Progressives recognized that corporate capitalism had brought about such an unprecedented concentration of economic and political power that it enabled employers to disregard consumer, child, and worker safety. Hence, "trust-busting," the breaking up of large commercial and industrial combines and monopolies, was part and parcel of the Progressive program. Virtually all the Progressives, especially Presidents Theodore Roosevelt and Woodrow Wilson, justified the dismantling of trusts to promote and restore faith in small entrepreneurship.

Progressives were not Socialist revolutionaries. On the contrary. Unlike socialism, Progressivism can be traced back to nineteenth-century laissez-faire theorists, who believed fervently in the opportunities provided by open markets and democratic politics. Despite their tendency to trust markets, in the early twentieth century Progressives came to believe that nineteenth-century opportunities had been exploited in the United States by a relatively small number of economic titans, "robber barons," whose power had corrupted political life and now threatened the very fabric of U.S. democracy. As a result, Progressives marshaled the power of the government itself, through popular ballot initiatives and legislation, to restore opportunity, equality, and social justice, all of which were necessary to ensure what they saw as the progress of U.S. civilization.[2]

Because of similar changes under way in Europe, French *solidaristes* shared many of these traits and political views.[3] Both countries were in the throes of large-scale industrialization, with its accompanying urbanization, social displacement, and concentration of economic power. As a result, class politics moved to the fore. Few now remember that the American Socialist Party received nearly a million votes, 6 percent of the total, in the U.S. presidential election of 1912. Because of France's multiparty parliamentary system, Socialists were even stronger, garnering one in six votes cast before 1914. Like their Progressive counterparts, *solidaristes* owed a debt to nineteenth-century European liberalism, which had inspired continentwide revolts against dynastic monarchs and the highly regulated economies over which they reigned.

Also like the Progressives, *solidaristes* represented an alternative to class warfare; they advocated commonsense compromises between socialism and unbridled capitalism. *Solidaristes* insisted that a new approach was needed to achieve the French republic's promise of equality; that the bourgeois conception of liberty as simply laissez-faire economics would result in social upheaval and revolution. The *solidariste* program was especially appealing after the First World War, which had proved much longer and deadlier than anyone had anticipated. To sustain popular support, wartime leaders had promised a postwar world of rights and prosperity. Such promises were mirrored in the United States in Wilsonian pledges of a more just society and a world "safe for democracy."

No single political party in either the United States or France had a monopoly on the Progressive or *solidariste* reform movements. Indeed, before 1912, Progressivism was closely associated with Republicans, fired by the party's western and midwestern leaders. Yet their enthusiasm for reform attracted few allies among the Republican establishment leaders in the Northeast. After a failed effort to create an autonomous Progressive Party to put Theodore Roosevelt back in the White House in 1912, Progressive constituents found a makeshift home in the more pluralistic Democratic Party, but no formal ties were ever envisioned.[4] Likewise, France's Radical Party claimed *solidarisme* as its own, but as a constituency, *solidaristes* were difficult to define. They tended to be middle-class voters who were restrained in their criticism of the status quo and rewarded any political leader who offered gradualist reform programs that promised stability. These potentially powerful Progressive and *solidariste* constituencies, combined with the trauma of industrialization, provided a wind at the back of reformers on both sides of the Atlantic. Socialists in both countries had long been advocates of government intervention in health care. But the issue reached new heights of visibility when Progressives and *solidaristes* placed it on their respective national agendas.

In the United States, the first Progressive efforts to create compulsory health insurance came from the American Association for Labor Legislation (AALL), founded in 1906. AALL leaders saw themselves as "a disinterested party mediating between the two poles of capital and labor," a sort of think tank without a financial stake in the legislation it proposed.[5] This was certainly true for the issue that catapulted the AALL to national prominence: the use of poisonous phosphorus by match manufacturers. Through investigatory research and an effective lobbying campaign in 1911, the AALL had convinced most members of Congress that the tooth loss and decomposing jawbones suffered by many match plant workers were directly linked to the use of phosphorus in the manufacturing process. In 1912 President Howard Taft signed into law a bill written by the AALL that banned the use of poisonous phosphorus. The case of phosphorus played to the strengths of the AALL leadership. Drawn almost exclusively from academia—primarily the University of Wisconsin, Yale, and Columbia—AALL leaders excelled at producing well-researched policy papers that guided legislators toward a desired political decision. The forces arrayed against them in the phosphorus case, namely match manufacturers, were relatively small and easily tagged as self-interested. Their battle for compulsory health insurance would prove much larger and more complex.

Like many Progressives of the era, AALL leaders looked to Europe for models, which in the case of health insurance meant primarily Britain and Germany. U.S. reformers preferred to tout the British system, especially after the United States entered the First World War in 1917. French social reformers, conversely, whose health insurance initiatives came immediately after the war, confronted a German system within their own borders. In victory, France regained territories in Alsace and Lorraine, which Germany had taken after its triumph in the 1870 Franco-Prussian War. Hence, in an ironic parallel, the Americans and the French were both inspired by their former enemies to take up health insurance reform—the United States by its onetime colonial master, Britain, France by its longtime nemesis, Germany.

British and German Models in the United States and France

In 1911 British lawmakers had approved the National Insurance Act (NIA), which paid medical care expenses and provided cash benefits for all wage earners, whether in factories, on the farm, or in domestic service. In exchange for their compulsory premiums, which made up 40 percent of NIA revenue, workers enjoyed twenty-six weeks of illness coverage, as well as disability and maternity benefits. Employers provided the remaining 60 percent of necessary revenues. The British system established an actuarial reserve, which over time paid the full price of a worker's illness during his or her life span. The actuarial soundness of British health insurance marked a departure from German-style social insurance, under which the premiums of healthy young workers covered the higher medical expenses and wage replacement stipends for their elder comrades. Today, the German approach is commonly referred to as "pay as you go." Britain's decision to create an actuarially sound insurance system stemmed from its choice to rely on the country's already numerous friendly societies as insurance carriers. Friendly societies were to Britain what mutual aid societies were to France and fraternal orders were to the United States: private insurance clubs that catered to solidly employed men. By emphasizing actuarial soundness, British lawmakers sought in advance to assure the solvency of local society funds, even in the absence of young recruits.[6]

British physicians had fought hard to enshrine their professional autonomy under the country's new compulsory health insurance. But they cared less about what most U.S. and French doctors considered indispensable to the practice of medicine, namely, patient choice and direct payment of fees. British physicians who wanted to participate in NIA signed onto regional panels. Beneficiaries enjoyed free choice of doctor but only from among those who had enrolled on their local panel. What is more, British physicians appreciatively accepted the payment of their fees from local insurance committees, a marked departure from the then-prevalent U.S. and French ethics regarding third-party payers who might violate doctor-patient confidentiality.

Within a few years of the NIA's passage, physicians with rural and working-class practices reported steep rises in income. Doctors who had previously been unable to collect any fees at all from their poor clientele emerged as the law's strongest backers. Indeed, from an ambivalent stance in 1911, the British medical profession propelled the NIA to success within seven years.[7] The British Medical Association's endorsement of compulsory health insurance had an especially significant influence on reformers and doctors in the United States.

Progressive AALL leaders, perched in their offices high above the streets of Manhattan, viewed the adoption of compulsory health insurance as a rational choice, not unlike the law they had written to ban noxious phosphorus from the workplace. Once the facts had been persuasively presented, they believed, most leaders, whether state legislators, AMA officials, union heads, or even employers in many cases, would line up in support. Like their campaign for industrial accident insurance, they believed victory would come quickly and decisively. During the first year of their effort, such a view appeared well founded.

The AALL chose a state-by-state strategy and quickly set out to draft legislation. Progressives believed that in the absence of ramifications for direct interstate commerce, the Constitution prevented them from seeking federal legislation on health insurance. Although passage in numerous state legislatures appeared cumbersome, they hoped that by succeeding in a few large states, similar legislation would easily pass elsewhere. A sort of domino effect of compulsory health insurance would sweep the country. This had been the case with earlier worker's compensation laws, and the AALL leaders hoped to repeat that success.

U.S. reformers had to settle on a name for their initiative. They called it "health insurance" rather than the more German "sickness insurance." But in reality, the AALL proposal was decidedly more Teutonic than English. Although the draft bill resembled the British NIA in professing to reach industrial, commercial, agricultural, and domestic workers, it defined beneficiaries as "every person employed in the state at manual labor under any form of wage contract." Thus, despite the bill's expressed intent, it actually excluded domestic workers, or, as the bill called them, "home workers and casual employees," many of whom were women, because they usually had no wage contracts. According to AALL leaders, women workers did not merit direct health security protections because women should be taken care of by what they consistently referred to as male "breadwinners."[8] These Ivy League social reformers surely knew that reliance on wage contracts for eligibility also automatically excluded most of the African American agricultural laborers south of the Mason-Dixon line, as well as farmworkers in the Southwest and California. Clearly, for the AALL, the most deserving citizens were white men employed under collective bargaining agreements in the manufacturing centers of the Northeast and Midwest.

For workers who could participate, the bill offered substantial benefits in exchange for light premiums: 1.6 percent of wages. Employers contributed the same proportion, while the state paid 0.8 percent, creating total revenues of 4 percent of wages. Like the German system, the draft bill envisioned local insurance funds as the "normal carrier."[9] The AALL bill permitted a variety of arrangements for medical services and cash benefits from which insurers could select. As in Britain, they could create a panel of doctors from which beneficiaries could choose, though no one physician could serve "more than 500 insured families nor more than 1,000 insured individuals." Payment for services rendered under this option would pass through a third-party insurer to physicians under a negotiated fee schedule or on a capitated basis. Alternatively, a local insurance fund could employ salaried physicians among whom "the insured persons shall have reasonable free choice."[10] Meanwhile, cash benefits under the AALL plan were quite generous: two-thirds of base pay for a maximum twenty-six weeks as well as substantial maternity benefits for women.

The AALL bill expressly recommended against the use of existing fraternal societies as insurance carriers. They explained that compulsory health insurance must rely on government-run carriers "until evidence is...brought forward to show that there exists a framework to voluntary societies, fraternals, trade unions, establishment benefit funds, strong enough and widely enough extended to support insurance." The unwillingness of AALL leaders to reach out to existing and potential private insurers dogged their effort from the beginning. In reply to their critics, AALL leaders claimed to be seeking the "most effective organization for combining employers and employees in a campaign for sickness prevention, and a most practical means for fixing rates and administering benefits."[11] If AALL leaders had expressed more appreciation of the individual's freedom to choose his existing fraternal order or union-run insurance fund, they would have outflanked many of their opponents.

Despite its shortcomings, the AALL plan found numerous supporters, especially in states where the Progressive movement was already strong. "Many wage earners, too proud to ask for charity treatment, get either no treatment at all, treatment too long delayed, or treatment of dubious value." So stated the U.S. Public Health Service in a 1916 pamphlet. The authors continued: "According to the experience in other countries as well as in the United States, private and commercial health insurance has failed to afford the relief and lighten the burden in the case of workers who stand in the greatest need."[12] In January 1917, a California state commission unanimously recommended the AALL draft bill to the state's legislature, nearly without change. Its findings underlined the political salience of government programs in favor of workers' health security. The commission noted: "The present laissez-faire method of ignoring the great problem of illness among wage earning families until actual destitution demands public attention, is social wasteful in the extreme."[13]

When the U.S. mobilization for the war in 1917 exposed far higher rates of poor health and disability among recruits than predicted, the AALL quickly cast compulsory health insurance as a way to repair a dangerous chink in the nation's armor—its young fighting men. The Massachusetts Insurance Commission unabashedly explored the tension between individual liberty and the common good of a well-regulated militia. Members clearly found that their discussion bore similarities to the debate over the AALL bill. Commissioners conceded that it was "natural" to view compulsory health insurance as "an un-American infringement of the principle of personal liberty." But they likened health insurance to one of the few issues where the need for compulsion was generally agreed on: national defense. "Every male citizen in Massachusetts between certain ages is by law a member of its militia. . . . Let it once be recognized clearly that every citizen has a duty to prepare himself to meet the hazards of life such as sickness, unemployment, and dependent old-age."[14] That a legislative proposal on health insurance could give rise to such far-reaching arguments indicates how close it cut to the nerve of contested U.S. values.

Whereas Progressives in the United States wished to portray their initiative as British, French reformers could not ignore the German model, a large piece of which their nation now possessed within its own borders due to the war. Inhabitants of Alsace-Lorraine participated in social insurance that had been created by Chancellor Otto von Bismarck in the 1880s. Reformers benefited from French political leaders' perception that a successful re-integration of Alsace-Lorraine into France necessitated a swift standardization of laws, including those that governed social welfare. Questions from the inhabitants about their place in postwar France became an especially urgent political issue immediately after the Armistice in 1918. An autonomist movement appeared as a potentially disruptive force in Alsace-Lorraine by 1919 and helped to focus the French government's attention on the transition from German to French rule.[15]

The potential loss of health insurance, which had been guaranteed under the German Reich, loomed among the most significant anxieties of Alsace-Lorraine's inhabitants. In meetings with workers' organizations in the months following the war, France's commissioner general, Alexandre Millerand, sought to reassure the region's inhabitants. He promised that "the three branches of your social insurance [health, disability, and old age] will be maintained in their entirety. . . . [France] will not only conserve the advantages enjoyed by the workers of Alsace-Lorraine under current legislation but will borrow appropriate elements of this legislation in order to improve its own laws and procure new benefits for all French workers."[16]

Health insurance funded through paycheck withholding and employer contributions was the oldest and most well established of the German social protections. Although the proportion of the population covered under Germany's health insurance was not as great as that under Britain's NIA, the law compelled most low- and moderate-income wage earners in industry and commerce to join. Others with incomes below a moderate threshold could enroll voluntarily. Counting insured dependents, approximately one-third of Alsace-Lorraine's population enjoyed health coverage. Medical care, including hospital stays and pharmaceuticals, were 100 percent covered for up to twenty-six weeks. Incapacitated workers also received an illness allowance of at least 50 percent of their base pay and half again that much in case of hospitalization. During an era when lost wages usually dwarfed medical expenses and a large proportion of the workforce had little or no savings, the illness allowance represented a critical component of health security. Fully 44 percent of expenditures at Alsace's Strasbourg insurance office went to illness allowances.[17]

What did physicians think of the German-style health insurance system under which they practiced? A postwar poll indicated that a vast majority favored maintaining compulsory health insurance and a clear majority believed that the system's "advantages outweighed its disadvantages." In 1922, the principal physicians' association in Alsace-Lorraine formally recommended compulsory health insurance to France's national doctors' association, the Union des Syndicats Médicaux de France (USMF).[18] But like British doctors under their new National Insurance Act, physicians in Alsace-Lorraine had embraced practices that most French doctors found anathema.

Foremost among these was the acceptance of a third-party payer. In a typical case, a worker selected a physician who agreed to treat him according to a fee schedule that had been negotiated between doctors and the social insurance office. Instead of billing a patient directly, doctors sent their bills to their local medical societies, where a small commission of their colleagues drew on an account provided by social insurance officials. Although itself created by the medical society, the payment commission had a financial motive to be severe with profligate doctors whose medical practices could not be justified.

After all, the commission's social insurance account had its limits. In practice, it could not exceed the combination of worker and employer contributions, which totaled 6 percent of wages. Government borrowing to pay for social welfare programs, now so common in the United States and France, was unheard of at the time. No doubt the commission may have been less scrupulous with local doctors when revenues were plentiful. But in periods of increased health care use, such as during the Spanish flu epidemic of 1918, the commission was forced to reduce payments to doctors. Physicians recognized these reductions as unfortunate but also noted that, on occasion, private patients did not pay at all. Their leaders were proud of their members' discipline, which they credited with permitting the negotiation of medical fees whose rates varied only slightly from those of the ordinary clientele.[19]

According to physicians in Alsace-Lorraine, German-style compulsory health insurance presented a danger to doctors only if they could not protect their sovereignty over medical decision making vis-à-vis insurers, that is, the state. If physicians were sufficiently united, they believed, doctors everywhere could confidently embrace the German model of health insurance to enhance coverage without endangering their profession.[20] Reports such as these heartened reformers in France and the United States.

In France, the first reform bill after World War I so closely resembled German health insurance that many must have wondered who had won the war. The Vincent bill, as it became known, called for the creation of regional insurance offices, which in turn negotiated contracts with local medical societies.[21] Hence, as in Germany, doctors were essentially contracted to provide medical services to local inhabitants under circumscribed conditions. Resistance from employers and mutual societies stymied the Vincent bill from its inception. It failed to reach a floor vote in the Chamber of Deputies; a Senate version was never even proposed. Nonetheless, its introduction created political momentum for compulsory health insurance that led to a second, more popular proposal by a physician-legislator, Edouard Grinda.

Grinda proclaimed that his bill represented a "social insurance [system], which is in essence a grand mutual society."[22] Workers obtained the new law's benefits through a mutual society of their choice or a government-run departmental fund, which quite often was directed by local mutual leaders. Indeed, Grinda's bill handed France's mutual societies a windfall of historic proportions. The bill provided coverage to low- and moderate-income industrial and commercial workers by levying a 2.5 percent wage tax that would be matched by employers. Spouses and dependent children of beneficiaries would also be covered, resulting in a total projected insured population of 9.3 million, or just under 25 percent of the total population.

On the specifics of medical practice, Grinda called for regional negotiations between insurers, be they mutual societies or departmental funds, and local medical societies, known as *syndicats*. The resulting contracts seemed to be limited only by the imaginations of the interlocutors; they could provide health care on capitated, fee-for-service, or hybrid bases. Even the possibility of salaried physicians who worked directly for mutual societies was not ruled out. Yet while reformers labored to draft viable legislation, employers on both sides of the Atlantic viewed the growing debate over compulsory health insurance as a high-stakes battle for control of their economic lives.

Employers and Paternalism

Employers argued that compulsory health insurance funded from their payrolls would lead to an unmitigated cataclysm. René Hubert of the French metals and mining industry characterized health insurance as "the greatest leap into the unknown" ever contemplated by a French legislature.[23] France's industrial trade press, beside itself with rage, called the proposal, "crazy...monstrous...a law of which one has to be ashamed."[24] Industrialist-backed trade publications in the United States were similarly outraged. The Associated Manufacturers and Merchants of New York called compulsory health insurance "as insane as anything that emanated from the wildest asylum in this country."[25]

Employers' more reasoned pronouncements raised two basic objections. The first concerned the effect on macroeconomic health. Daniel Ryan, general counsel for the Ohio Manufacturer's Association, found the "time inopportune for financial reasons to launch a system of social insurance."[26] One of France's best-known industrialists, René Duchemin, noted that insurance premiums would abet price increases in manufacturing, resulting in a "truly perilous threat to the workings of the national economy."[27] In both cases, employers predicted an inflationary spiral induced by social insurance that would hurt workers' real wages and threaten their ability to compete in world markets. For all the plausibility of such arguments, employers' actions betray a second, more pressing motive.

Control of nonwage compensation, especially medical care, had historically been a tool employers used to assuage and pacify their labor forces, what historians call "welfare capitalism" or "paternalism." If compulsory health insurance were enacted, medical care as a lever to control sometimes unwieldy workers would become ineffective. The First World War had led to a massive rise in union membership, as workers flooded the munitions factories to meet the demand for war materiel. After the Armistice, large portions of the U.S. and French labor forces engaged in strikes, which rocked the economies of both nations. Add to this news of the Communist revolution in Russia. The result was an intense effort on the part of industrialists to maintain control of their workers, which included providing medical care through the workplace. In the late 1910s and early 1920s, industrialists either directly employed company doctors or provided employer-funded benefits.

Company doctors were usually found in heavy industry, at railway companies, or in firms with far-flung workplaces, such as U.S. timber firms in the Pacific Northwest. These employers built clinics and hired company physicians to care for their workers. Some also employed surgeons who could quickly come to the aid of victims of all-too-common serious accidents. The railways made use of their ability to cheaply transport physicians and patients along their networks.[28] The Pacific Lumber Company built an entire town, Scotia, California, from the ground up, complete with company store, scrip, schools, and, of course, a company clinic and doctors. Even in the heartland, company-provided medicine made sense to large industrialists. In 1925, the United States Steel Corporation directly employed 225 physicians and surgeons and 251 nurses to provide medical care to its workers. Even smaller firms, such as Kodak, employed full-time doctors and nurses, and had eye and dental clinics.[29] France's Michelin Corporation adopted similar tactics. It owned a full array of medical facilities, including pharmacies, clinics, diagnostic centers, and hospitals providing health care to workers and their families. Michelin also built company housing, organized sports leagues, and paid generous family allowances to workers with dependent children. What was needed, insisted Michelin's director of social services, was not compulsory health insurance but "more clinics, dispensaries, maternal care, hospitals, spas, and sanatoria."[30] Of course, Michelin owned just such facilities in large numbers.

Industrial firms such as Michelin and United States Steel hoped to persuade their legislators that the achievements of employer-provided health care were reason enough to abandon plans for compulsory health insurance. Yet employer programs on this scale were also those most despised by workers. They suspected that management used company medical personnel to weed out workers, not just on physical grounds, but based on behavioral traits and political views. To combat this charge, Michelin responded with propaganda that likened state-directed health care to an assembly line: all workers would receive the same prescription despite their different ailments.

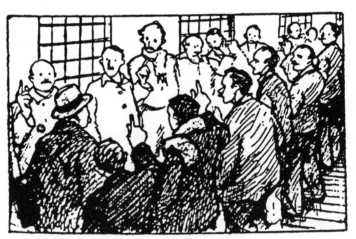

La consultation en série.
— Que les « mal de gorge » lèvent la main.

Figure 1. Illustration appearing in a 1927 Michelin pamphlet that extols the company's medical services and attacks government care as "assembly-line" treatment. The caption reads: "Assembly-line examinations—'Everybody with a sore throat raise your hand.'" "Oeuvres Sociales de Michelin et Cie" (Paris: Clermont-Ferrand, 1927).

U.S. and French workers' unions preferred employer-provided benefit funds to company doctors. In the United States, these funds took the form of voluntary mutual benefit associations, under which employers shared the cost of health insurance premiums with their workers and paid the full cost of fund administration. Such arrangements caused far less resentment among workers and union leaders while providing employers with a modicum of employee loyalty and better labor relations. Benefits varied widely, but a worker could typically count on a wage replacement stipend of about half his or her wages for ten to thirteen weeks of long-term incapacitation. In 1917, however, as the debate over the AALL bill heated up, only about 10 percent of U.S. industrial firms maintained mutual benefit associations that covered medical care or wage loss. For women and racial and ethnic minorities, the rates were much lower. In a 1914 survey of fourteen mutual benefit plans in New York, eight were closed to women altogether; the remaining four served only those women who qualified as wives or unmarried daughters of male members. African American workers suffered a similar fate. Mutual benefit associations were nearly nonexistent in agriculture and rare in industrial concerns where blacks were employed.[31]

French employers also maintained sickness insurance funds. Some, like the Renault automobile company, created company-run mutual aid societies, which were essentially similar to U.S. employers' mutual benefit associations. Yet French employers' most promising alternative to compulsory health insurance was neither company doctors nor mutual societies funded by employers. It involved a direct alliance between industrialists and private physicians, a model that is worthy of our sustained attention because it bolstered private-practice medicine and exposed fundamental problems regarding the reliance on employers for health security.

The largest of France's employer-physician alliances was the 1924 agreement in the northern textile-manufacturing region of Roubaix-Tourcoing.[32] The Roubaix-Tourcoing agreement brought area physicians a substantial patient load from a consortium of textile manufacturers, with only minor changes to the procedures they followed for other clients. Workers could select any doctor from the doctors' *syndicat*, which, in practice, meant any local practitioner. Patients were responsible for the full payment of their doctor's fees and sought reimbursement from their employers. Roubaix-Tourcoing textile manufacturers also provided a small stipend to replace lost wages, but it could not be collected unless the worker's incapacitation lasted more than eight days.

For French doctors, the alliance with employers furthered the cause of private-practice medicine: free choice of physician, medical confidentiality, freedom of diagnosis and therapy, and most important, the direct payment of fees. All were accepted by the textile manufacturers. In the words of one physician, this is "not a chimera: it exists, it works, it is progress. The truth is that French employers have shown the way for the whole world."[33] The freedoms afforded to doctors under these agreements aided in the negotiation of eighteen such contracts in industrial centers throughout the country, including Paris, Lille, Lyons, Saint-Etienne, and Grenoble.[34] Because dependents were included, the number of beneficiaries reached well into the millions by the mid-1920s. In Roubaix-Tourcoing alone, 250,000 employees and dependents were covered. Industrialists who offered medical benefits clearly hoped to create an alternative to compulsory health insurance, and a significant number of doctors enthusiastically cheered them on. "The more contracts of this type that are passed throughout France, the stronger will be our position," proclaimed a leader of the Roubaix medical *syndicat*.[35]

Nevertheless, an equally outspoken group of French physicians opposed employer health benefits as a deception, a short-term maneuver by industrialists, who, once the political momentum for compulsory health insurance had passed, would drop or reduce benefits as quickly as they had offered them.[36] These doctors argued that only a strong national doctors' association that engaged the government as a partner could assure an advantageous position for doctors while improving health care quality and access. These adversaries of employer-reliant health security found their most articulate spokesperson in René Lafontaine, a Parisian doctor and member of the governing board of the Union des Syndicats des Médecins de France (USMF), France's national federation of medical *syndicats*.

Lafontaine's attack on employer-based health care centered on the relatively powerless position of worker-beneficiaries, whom he distinguished from properly empowered insurees. The beneficiary, Lafontaine bemoaned, "is that of a charity case, not of an insuree, an insuree possesses rights...a beneficiary has none. The beneficiary...does not participate in contract negotiations, he is an object; he has no voice."[37] To be sure, the principal drawbacks of the system for both patients and doctors flowed directly from beneficiaries' weakness. Employers enjoyed discretion to raise or lower their reimbursement of patients or to cancel benefits altogether. Thus, doctors and patients alike were at the mercy of industrialists' financial calculations: health security might be cut in the face of falling profits, a stagnant economy, or unemployment. Lafontaine's fears in this regard were underlined by employers' refusal to provide hospitalization, radiology, or long-term illness benefits. If an employee were sick enough to require these services, employers presumably judged that he or she would not be returning to work anytime soon. Employers preferred instead to make occasional donations to local charity hospitals that cared for the chronically ill; but patients there could no longer be considered beneficiaries of the employer-physician alliance—let alone workers.

This aspect of the employer-physician alliances precipitated a sharp (and edifying) public exchange between Lafontaine and the Roubaix doctors' *syndicat* leader Desrousseaux at a 1925 national medical meeting. Lafontaine queried his colleague about serious illnesses: "What do you do in cases when the patient needs to be hospitalized?" Desrousseaux could only respond with implausible denial: "We attach minimal importance to hospitalization because our people don't go to the hospital."[38] Even for short-term ambulatory care, employers held extraordinary powers of arbitration. Under the terms of the Roubaix-Tourcoing alliance, for example, neither patients nor doctors were empowered to initiate complaints; only the textile employers could do so. Since most complaints would presumably pertain to incompetent care or unjust reimbursement, this provision gagged unpleasant criticisms of the system from its two most likely sources: patients and doctors.

For Lafontaine, the spread of employer-based health benefits would result in the creation of two sorts of doctors. The first would remain in private practice, treating only patients with minor afflictions who had no recourse in the event of bad care and no access to long-term care for chronic conditions. The second would work in hospitals, specializing in the treatment of the seriously and chronically ill and the gravely injured. The future of those in the first category would be livable "but not brilliant, financially or ethically." As for the second, "they would become simple government employees," a status widely despised by French doctors.[39]

In their day, France's employer-physician alliances constituted a viable voluntary alternative to compulsory health insurance, one that left administrative control in the hands of employers and medical decision making in the hands of physicians. It thereby preserved many of the liberties that employers, patients, and doctors hoped to protect as medical care reached larger portions of the population. Despite these appeals, Lafontaine's critique of employer-physician alliances found broad sympathy among his fellow physicians, workers, and union leaders. Indeed, he raised the fundamental questions to which all employment-based health care systems must still answer. What rights should be guaranteed to workers who are also patients? What powers can employers who pay for their workers' medical care rightfully retain? And what role must government play to assure a balance between the two? As we look back nearly a century later, the prescience of Lafontaine's query is difficult to deny. During the first debates in the United States and France over compulsory health insurance, even labor leaders in both countries disagreed on the answers to his questions.

Unions' Disagreement over Health Care

U.S. workers' unions split over the AALL's compulsory health insurance proposal because they were unable to find any common ground between the competing ideals of individual liberty and interdependent citizenship or to agree on the proper role of the state in reconciling the two. France's unions also split over compulsory health insurance, but theirs was more an intraclass struggle for power and worker allegiance rather than a debate over the nation's founding principles. Divided though they were over how close to align themselves with Communist leaders in Soviet Russia, the rivalry between France's Socialist and Communist unions proved far less disruptive to health care reformers seeking working-class support.

Given the U.S. labor movement's lengthy and sometimes violent struggle against government repression, it is understandable that the leader of the American Federation of Labor (AFL), Samuel Gompers, looked with such deep suspicion on any proposal to empower state officials to control health care. Yet the AFL's rebuke of compulsory insurance stood just as firmly on the grounds of voluntarism and individualism; the AFL was unwilling even to accept the state as an equal partner with workers' unions. Gompers attacked the AALL's draft bill for its corrosive effect on the "independence of spirit."[40] The AFL newspaper, *The American Federationist,* noted that "social insurance...would substitute a paternalistic regime for...individual responsibility and freedom." The union thus rejected any government role in health insurance just as vehemently as it did employers' company doctors, even resorting to the term "paternalistic," usually reserved for invasive employers.

In one important sense, then, the AFL's opposition to compulsory health insurance differed little from employers'. The union sought to fend off a legislative solution to insufficient medical care and illness-induced poverty by creating voluntary associations of its own. Again, the AFL's *Federationist* noted: "Proposals to force upon the workers social insurance of compulsory nature have now taken such shape that unless the wage-earners protect themselves and establish their own devices, they will find themselves over-whelmed by state regulation and administration."[41] Without a doubt, the AFL's sickness insurance funds were more democratic organizations than industrialists' mutual benefit associations. But the AFL's rejection of com-pulsory health insurance set adrift millions of wage earners whose unions were incapable of sustaining a viable health insurance fund because of their inability to negotiate employer contributions or because of their concen-trated risk pools.

The AFL's opposition to compulsory health insurance also used a gen-dered notion of the deserving U.S. worker. When Gompers cited the cor-rosive effect of compulsory health insurance on individualism, he also warned of "a weakening of virility."[42] Women did not fit Gompers's no-tion of independent, deserving workers. In his view, women should remain dependent on virile men, who would create their own union-based insur-ance funds for the benefit of their families. Pauline Newman, leader of the 150,000-strong International Ladies Garment Workers' Union, challenged Gompers, proclaiming: "I do not call [state action] paternalism, because I am looking forward to the time when the state will come to the con-clusion that it owes something to its working men and women."[43] Many other labor leaders agreed with her. By 1919, the AALL had obtained the endorsement of dozens of state federations, including New York's, and of independent unions around the country, including the powerful United Mine Workers of America.[44] Despite this support, the AFL's early condem-nation of compulsory health insurance as a violation of individual liberty proved extremely damaging to reformers. Precisely because French unions did not split over such a core value, those who opposed compulsory health insurance in France proved far less harmful to reform.

Leaders of France's Communist trade union, the Confédération Géné-rale du Travail Unitaire (CGTU) opposed the Grinda bill on compulsory health insurance, but for very different reasons than those of the AFL. They believed that compulsory social insurance was a trick foisted on the work-ing class to delay the day of Communist revolution. Writing in the Com-munist daily, L'Humanité, Félix Paoli insisted that the legislation "will only be a law of appeasement, refusing, as always, the social justice for which we have fought and will not see until there is a total transformation of the economy."[45] Yet as strong as the Communists were in France at the time, their opposition counted for much less than the AFL's in the United States. The Communists spoke with less historical legitimacy than their Socialist rivals on ideals that were central to the debate over compulsory health insurance.

France's Socialist Party and its associated trade union, the Confédération Générale du Travail (CGT), claimed a heritage that hearkened back to the Jacobin egalitarianism of the French Revolution. Jacobins had led France's First Republic during its most violent phase, but nineteenth-century Socialists, especially Jean Jaurès (1859–1914), had successfully transformed France's Jacobin-fired egalitarian Left into a unified Social Democratic party that was committed to democracy and individual liberty. To be sure, of France's revolutionary triptych, "Liberté, Egalité, Fraternité," the Socialists' political agenda emphasized the latter two terms. But in contrast to their Communist rivals, the Socialists' acceptance of the French Republic, and their status in Parliament, made them important allies of France's *solidaristes* in the battle for compulsory health insurance. As one CGT official put it, "I don't see myself as a fan of this parliament… but it must be said, the Grinda bill constitutes an important development that can be accepted as a basis for social insurance in our country."[46]

Unlike AFL leaders, who rejected ties to the American Socialist Party and openly attacked Progressives' health care initiative by insisting on worker autonomy and voluntarism at all cost, the Socialist CGT embraced interdependent citizenship and compulsion—a position that left its Communist rivals on the sidelines. By the mid-1930s, Socialists had so outpaced Communists that they could lead a government without them, turning instead to the *solidariste*-dominated Radical Party as allies. The Socialist CGT's position also benefited from the small but not insignificant third leg of France's trade union movement, the Social Catholic Confédération Française des Travailleurs Chrétiens (CFTC). Hence, in contrast to the difficulties of American Progressives, French *solidaristes* were far better positioned to build a multipartisan compromise across class lines in favor of compulsory health insurance. When insurers and doctors entered the fray, debates in both countries reached their climax.

Fraternal Orders, Mutual Aid Societies, and Commercial Insurers

Insurers had much at stake in the debate over compulsory health insurance. In the United States, reformers angered leaders of the nation's fraternal movement, driving them into an unlikely alliance with their rivals, the commercial insurance companies. Meanwhile, because of France's more expansive mutual aid movement, commercial insurers had little voice in the debate over compulsory health insurance. Yet despite their favorable treatment under the Grinda bill, mutual leaders split over whether mutual societies should accept the hand proffered by legislators, thereby becoming principal carriers under the new law.

U.S. fraternal orders were suspicious of government-sponsored health insurance from the beginning. Their newspaper, the *Fraternal Monitor,* labeled it inimical to "that spirit of self-reliance so essential for continued progress and prosperity."[47] Worse still, the AALL had included a funeral benefit in its proposal that would have undermined the sale of similar protections by fraternal orders. This led many fraternal leaders to wonder whether the AALL was a friend or a foe. When AALL leaders held fast to the funeral benefit, most fraternal leaders concluded that the answer was "foe." Some believed their very existence was at stake, that "the protection of several million people in voluntary societies will become unnecessary and cease to exist."[48] Distrust of the AALL's intentions sent the fraternal movement headlong toward the opposing forces where, ironically, they sided with increasingly powerful commercial insurers, who had designs of their own on fraternal orders.

Until the 1920s, the insurance industry, led by Equitable, Metropolitan, and Prudential, had divided up the life insurance market, selling individual policies, often door-to-door. In exchange for a flat low monthly premium, most policies paid a modest burial fee and a onetime indemnity that ranged between 25 and 100 percent of the insured's annual wages. It was in this market that fraternal orders and commercial insurers, especially Metropolitan, competed for working-class subscribers.

The fact that the AALL's draft bill had been inspired by European models of social insurance horrified life insurance executives. Equitable's president told his staff, "Insurance by the state is neither desirable nor necessary in this land of the greatest life insurance corporations the world has ever known."[49] But it was Metropolitan that launched the most effective counterattack on compulsory health insurance. First, the company moved aggressively into the group life insurance market, targeting new working-class subscribers through their employers. Next, Metropolitan's president, Haley Fiske, recruited Lee Frankel, a well-known Progressive reformer with ties to the AALL. Frankel reinvented the company's Welfare Division, launching programs that focused on workers' health. He held picnics, sponsored a visiting-nurse program, distributed health education pamphlets, and provided free medical exams. Frankel's initiatives fit perfectly with the new scientific approaches to manufacturing and mass production then being advocated by Frederick Winslow Taylor. This collusion of interests, rationale, and effort among employers and group life insurers laid the foundations for a new generation of employer-based welfare benefits, including health coverage.

It is critical to note that prior to the AALL's campaign for compulsory health insurance, commercial insurers had shown little interest in medical matters. Indeed, throughout the history of health care, the mere prospect of government intervention has repeatedly determined the timing if not the nature of private sector action. The AALL's early momentum in 1916 prompted commercial insurers to develop a health insurance benefit of their own to prove that government compulsion was not required.

Metropolitan's Lee Frankel condemned his former AALL colleagues and compulsory health insurance altogether.[50] Moreover, he and his fellow commercial insurers' take-no-prisoners counterattack reveals that they contemplated no possibility of compromise even if the AALL had withdrawn the funeral benefit, something that state legislators were free to do in any case. Commercial insurers believed that the success of compulsory health insurance would "bring about the result that all forms of insurance—life, casualty, fire and every other form—shall be carried solely by the government."[51] For commercial insurers, nothing less than their entrepreneurial liberties were at stake.

To match Metropolitan's Lee Frankel, Prudential employed Frederick Hoffmann, another former AALL Progressive. Hoffman had been a key supporter of the AALL's campaign against match manufacturers' use of poisonous phosphorous. Yet he objected to the AALL's health insurance initiative because it excluded commercial insurance companies as carriers. Because Hoffman was a well-established expert on industrial accidents and disease, he could escape being tagged a self-serving spokesperson of commercial insurers.[52] Toward this end, Hoffman made ample use of statistics. He sought to show, for example, that "the existing amount of ill health in American industry is not excessive" enough to warrant a compulsory system that would lead to an "annual income loss of $800,000,000." As a German-American living during the First World War, Hoffman also found it prudent to attack the effectiveness of German health insurance. In a typical tract, he called attention to greater progress in the United States in reducing tuberculosis deaths and the country's higher life expectancy, which led him to conclude that it "is therefore absurd to argue that the wage-earners of this country are suffering physical deterioration." Of course, the AALL's plan primarily sought to ameliorate the health security of workers, not rescue them from "physical deterioration." Nevertheless, Hoffman's reputation and angle of attack led state health commissions to summon him to testify before them, not as a spokesperson of commercial insurers but as an expert witness. Hoffman's use of this platform proved extremely damaging to the AALL's campaign, especially when, at the end of his expert testimony, he pronounced that "compulsion or coercion in matters of social reform is antagonistic to our American conceptions of personal freedom in a democracy."[53] Hoffman further insisted that compulsory health insurance was unbefitting "citizenship of a free republic," knowing full well that the largest European republic and U.S. ally, France, had, at least until that time, opted for voluntary solutions when it came to health security.[54]

Together with fraternal orders and employers, commercial insurers also funded umbrella organizations to fight the AALL. These included the Insurance Economics Society of America and the National Civic Federation. Suffering from a tarnished public image that diminished their claim to speak for the common good, commercial insurers preferred to work through such umbrella groups. A scandal at Equitable early in the century and repeated revelations by the muckraking press of lavish salaries for insurance executives reinforced these perceptions. Such was not the case in France, where commercial insurers were far less prevalent, leaving the mutual movement to speak for insurers in the debate over compulsory health insurance.

In contrast to commercial insurers in the United States, French mutual societies enjoyed an unsullied reputation of public service. But that does not mean they did not fight over whether to support compulsory health insurance. After all, France's mutual movement was the institutional embodiment of the nation's voluntarist instinct, which emphasized liberty and self-help over social welfare, traits that could not be easily suppressed. A mutual leader from Normandy, Henri Vermont, led the foes of compulsory insurance, calling it "German," the era's most slanderous epithet. Vermont further insisted that its passage would reduce mutual societies to nothing more than bureaucratic ancillaries of the state.[55]

In the midst of Vermont's attack, France's influential *solidariste* legislators, whose connections to the mutual movement ran deep, succeeded in elevating two of their own, Raoul Péret and Georges Petit, to the leadership of the nation's mutual federation, the Fédération Nationale de la Mutualité Française.[56] In a savvy political maneuver, Petit openly challenged legislators to give mutual societies a chance to demonstrate their expertise and commitment to social insurance: "Mr. Minister, I must say, we've had enough. If you want social insurance, vote on it. . . . 'The rail car has been placed on the tracks.' We're good engineers and we'll take responsibility for driving that train to a happy destination."[57] This put mutual leaders who opposed social insurance in the position of shying away from a challenge that Petit had openly accepted. Petit also pressed mutual societies to use their cash reserves to build clinics, pharmacies, and hospitals, and sought looser government regulations that would permit them to become major health care providers. Together, these policies positioned France's mutual movement better than even the most optimistic proponents of compulsory health insurance had hoped. Indeed, they signaled that most mutual leaders would support compulsory health insurance as long as the law incorporated their societies as partners.[58]

This tactic stands in stark contrast to that of U.S. fraternal orders and commercial insurers. Instead of writing themselves into the law, they fought it, convinced that compulsory health insurance was a wedge for the government's takeover of all insurance services. Their alliance with employers and AFL leader Gompers created a formidable wall of resistance against U.S. reformers.

Doctors of the Right, Left, and Center

Like the French mutual movement, physicians initially split over the issue of compulsory health insurance. Advocates of reform dominated the early stages of the debate, but as more physicians participated, prospects for reform faded. In France, compulsory health insurance bills became so hotly contested that the national doctors' confederation, the USMF, broke into rival camps. In the United States, the American Medical Association (AMA) avoided an organizational schism but suffered a divisive struggle that lasted into the early 1920s.

Both the French and U.S. medical associations broke into three distinct factions. Advocates favored compulsory insurance but insisted on the freedom of local medical societies to negotiate whatever contract they deemed appropriate with local health insurance authorities. They faced off against conservatives who opposed any government intervention that would compel the purchase of insurance. In between were centrist groups, whose compromise positions gained credence only late in the debate. Centrists accepted the principle of compulsion as long as physicians maintained broad control over medical decision making and doctor-patient relations. In France, the centrists triumphed. In the United States, conservatives turned back reformers' early momentum and avoided a centrist compromise. Yet these contrasting political outcomes should not mask a critical similarity. In both nations, private-practice medicine emerged as the sole legitimate form of medical practice, a development that would have repercussions every bit as important as the different decisions about compulsory health insurance.

The Union des Syndicats Médicaux de France (USMF) suffered the most from French doctors' internecine strife over compulsory health insurance. Up until this time, doctors' political energies had remained focused on matters closer to home. Local medical *syndicats* dealt directly with regional employers, mutual societies, and charity institutions, which required collective relations with physicians. Legislative deliberations over compulsory health insurance inevitably thrust the union into the national spotlight as a critical interlocutor with legislators and government officials. When the first health insurance bill was introduced in 1921, the USMF enrolled fifteen thousand members out of a total medical corps of twenty-three thousand. The union's single largest group hailed from its Paris *syndicat*, which alone possessed a membership of over a thousand.[59] Membership in the USMF rose quickly in the early 1920s once its pivotal role in legislative lobbying became apparent. But what seemed a ready-made vehicle for expressing physicians' collective interest vis-à-vis the government soon became a showcase of disunity.[60]

In the United States, on the eve of the campaign over health insurance in 1915, the AMA's membership, as a percentage of the nation's doctors, was much lower than its French counterpart. Only about half of all doctors thought it necessary to belong, despite the fact that the AMA had successfully reorganized itself in the early years of the century. A new House of Delegates elected by county medical societies through state representatives replaced the previously cumbersome organization, which had allotted power to various groups such as medical colleges, state medical societies, and hospitals. The reorganization also created a national headquarters in Chicago where an executive council and board of trustees met to carry out the will of the House of Delegates and to play a greater role in public policy deliberations.

When the Progressive movement swept the country, AMA leaders applauded, supporting the Pure Food and Drug Act, a national health department, as well as government subsidies for medical education, as long as the subsidies did not threaten the professional autonomy of physician training.[61] In fact, the AMA's turn-of-the-century reorganization translated into early support from the medical profession for compulsory health insurance. The AMA's executive council and staff exhibited decidedly

Progressive leanings. They tended to view European models of compulsory health insurance as alluring, and, in some cases, inevitable.

Before long, however, the Progressive-leaning leaders at AMA headquarters in Chicago found themselves in open conflict with conservative opponents in state medical societies. Instead of seeking to influence legislation, conservatives created a vision of entrepreneurial freedom, prestige, and professional sovereignty in which compulsory health insurance had no role whatsoever. The result was a fractious battle within the AMA that included nationalistic appeals and intimidation. The winners set the course for the U.S. medical profession on health insurance and defined permissible forms of medical practice for much of the rest of the century.

Meanwhile, proreform doctors in both countries embraced a remarkably similar line of reasoning. They viewed the advent of compulsory health insurance as inevitable because of larger socioeconomic change, namely, industrialization and urbanization. Reformers also believed that physicians should be proactive, not reactive, to societal change. In 1910, the AMA's flagship publication, the *Journal of the American Medical Association*, editorialized, "American physicians should be so well organized that the [compulsory health insurance] laws would prove a blessing rather than a curse and this could be best accomplished by joining a revitalized AMA." Just as the AALL campaign was getting under way in 1916, the *Medical Record* likewise counseled, "Whether one likes it or not, social health insurance is bound to come sooner or later, and it behooves the medical profession to meet this condition with dignity. . . . Blind condemnation will lead nowhere."[62]

In a similar vein, French physicians who advocated compulsory insurance insisted that, with or without doctors, health insurance would become law. Their leader, René Lafontaine, was the same doctor who criticized the power of employers over health care. He dismissed as obsolete the views of opponents who condemned health insurance because they "wish only to see individuals." This, he charged, was confusing the value of individualized medicine, which he too prized, with the role that physicians must play to protect it. Lafontaine warned that the "artisan [had] disappeared; he became a [factory] worker. . . . Will we one day be compelled to become wage-earning workers in organizations . . . where bankers . . . play the leading role?" Unlike factory workers, he continued, "We are the masters of medicine; we can negotiate conditions under which neither the provision of medical care nor its providers are subordinated to anonymous power." In other words, Lafontaine believed that physicians' scientific and technical know-how could save them from professional extinction, but only if they had a powerful, unified association. Compulsory health insurance thus offered doctors a historic opportunity to disconnect medical care delivery from employers and insurers and to bolster physicians' control, but only if they acted in unison and at once, "*when the organization is being created.*"[63]

Conservatives, meanwhile, appealed to national character to attack reformers. In so doing, conservatives often painted proreform physicians as somehow "un-American" or "un-French," blatantly calling their patriotism into question. This was especially true in the United States after April 1917, when the country entered the war against Germany. Conservative detractors simply ignored the fact that Britain, a U.S. ally, had just instituted compulsory insurance, focusing instead on the enemy, Germany. "What is Compulsory Social Health Insurance?" asked California's conservative League for the Conservation of Public Health, which replied: "It is a dangerous device, invented in Germany, announced by the German Emperor from the throne in the same year he started plotting and preparing to conquer the world."[64] Such polemics created a climate that made it possible to intimidate anyone who might back compulsory health insurance, especially those who happened to have German ancestry.

In his 1918 AMA presidential address, Arthur Dean Bevan warned his audience: "We as a profession must go into this war not only efficient, but we must go into it 100 percent loyal, 100 percent American....There are a few [physicians] who are disloyal and would give aid and comfort to the enemy, these must be sought out and interned where they can do no harm." A pamphlet by a New York dermatologist called proreform physicians "crypto-Bolsheviks" and claimed that Socialism would be "as firmly established by compulsory health insurance as it would be by the acceptance of the whole Marxian system."[65] Out of fear, self-censorship became the rule. At a Pennsylvania medical conference, one participant asked who supported compulsory health insurance. The presiding officer responded that it surely was not the medical profession because "no one had found a real, live, practicing medical man to speak a word on its behalf." Meanwhile, Doctor F. L. Van Sickle, who barely two years earlier had authored the Pennsylvania State Medical Society's endorsement of the AALL bill, sat in the audience but chose to say nothing.[66]

The association made between compulsory health insurance and foreign agents, especially Communist revolutionaries in Russia, complemented warnings from the AFL and from employers about the initiative's destructive effect on liberty and individual responsibility. Indeed, by 1919 the two arguments had become one. What had once been a respected if not universally accepted U.S. notion of community spirit and fair play was now equated with Russian Communism. Even the staid language of a committee report to the Ohio state legislature insists that if employers and workers were compelled to share the risk of illness it would "place upon society as a whole...the responsibility for individual failure" and "bring us dangerously close to policies which are at present of the gravest concern to the entire civilized world," a clear reference to the Bolsheviks.[67] According to such reasoning, the individual must bear risks alone or search out voluntary means of protection. What was left unsaid was that much of the U.S. labor force had no opportunity to join or create voluntary associations against the risks of ill health because of their race or gender, or because of professional barriers.

Physician backers of health insurance in France were quite familiar with the scorn heaped on U.S. reformers who advocated German-style social protections. Since the nineteenth century, most political leaders and social commentators had proudly regarded voluntarism and individual self-help in democratic France as in fitting contrast to the compulsory nature of social welfare in imperial Germany. Even on pressing public health issues of hygiene or the quarantine of victims of highly contagious diseases, where scientific evidence fell overwhelmingly on the side of compulsion, proponents of forceful state action were summarily dismissed as dangerously Teutonic and out of touch with what it meant to be French. France, it was said, was the cradle of *liberté*; its people could never submit to a system that compelled individuals to forgo personal choice on matters as important as illness and medicine.[68]

French proreform physicians, however, were greatly aided by the return of Alsace-Lorraine to France. Because of the popularity of German social insurance in Alsace-Lorraine, national leaders who insisted on uniformity and equity across the republic had no choice but to consider reforms for the rest of the country. Unlike in the United States, where the Revolutionary War had resulted in a federal system of constitutionally protected states' rights, France's revolution culminated in Napoleon's rise to power. Napoleon committed himself to the French Revolution's gains at the expense of aristocratic privilege and excess, yet he also created a highly centralized administrative state, surpassing even that achieved by previous French monarchs. Since Napoleon, departmental prefects selected in Paris—not elected from the departments where they served—had propagated uniform national policies, including those concerned with education and health.

Yet national uniformity mattered little to conservative French physicians such as André Jayle, who opposed compulsory health insurance throughout the 1920s. Jayle believed that compulsory health insurance violated the natural disposition of the French. His arguments used the eugenic rhetoric of the time, simply recasting the appeal to individual self-help and responsibility so common in the United States in pseudoscientific language. Compulsory health insurance, Jayle insisted, was "dangerous for humanity.... The strong and solid...pay for the sickly and weak.... The result is to overburden the strong who, from the eugenic perspective, must run society." Moreover, Jayle continued, such insurance ran contrary to what it meant to be French because it was based on "German thinking." He conceded that it might work for Germans because they were "disciplined through force." But it would prove disastrous in France where "one only accepts the discipline imposed by oneself."[69] Jayle would have allowed the continuation of compulsory health insurance in Alsace-Lorraine. But French doctors, which in his view clearly did not include his Alsatian colleagues, could not stoop to participate in compulsory health insurance. "Just as doctors are not the same everywhere, French doctors are superior to others. Just as the human races are not equal...France is in no way behind other peoples concerning social insurance."[70] Jayle's underlying premise that what was German could not also be French struck a resonant cord among physicians and the broader public,[71] as did the notion that compulsory health insurance represented a Bolshevik wedge in French society. Opponents shouted accusations of "Bolshevik! Soviet!" at proponents, who replied with equally caustic jibes of "Dictator!"[72] Amidst of it all in both countries, moderate physicians wondered whether a compromise among the warring factions was possible. In France, the rise of this third group under the mantle of private-practice medicine portended a major divergence in the health care systems of the two nations.

France's centrist group was headed by the mercurial Paul Cibrie, who ran the Paris medical *syndicat*. Cibrie accepted the idea of compulsory health insurance, but only if it embraced unconditional protections of fee-for-service private-practice medicine and physicians' unquestioned clinical freedoms. The centrists' triumph in France was due in large part to Cibrie's remarkable political skills and the allure with which he painted private medicine as an exclusive model for general practitioners and specialists alike. Early in the debate, Cibrie more often than not sided with René Lafontaine, who viewed employer-provided health care as vastly more dangerous to doctors than any government-directed compulsory insurance. In alliance with Lafontaine, Cibrie built a reputation as an able spokesperson for the interests of Paris physicians, most of whom shared Lafontaine's concern about employer-provided medical benefits and appreciated his advocacy of strong medical *syndicats*.

As the debate reached its height, however, Cibrie broke with Lafontaine, developing a doctrine of his own. In contrast to the conservative Jayle, Cibrie accepted the government's role in compelling workers and employers to pay for health insurance. But in exchange for doctors' participation in compulsory health insurance, he insisted that employers, insurers, and the government must respect physicians' professional sovereignty and the unique legitimacy of fee-for-service medicine. Cibrie's position appealed to conservatives who had supported Jayle as well as to proreform doctors who had backed Lafontaine. To conservatives, Cibrie offered a comforting view of physician autonomy drawn from an idealized notion of medical practice where insurers and employers had no influence. Yet the independence that Cibrie wished for the physician remained circumscribed by the principles of fee-for-service private-practice medicine, on which Cibrie was unyielding. He condemned all other arrangements, including capitated payments and salaried physicians, as "immoral."[73]

In the United States, Eden V. Delphey, a New York general practitioner, adopted a similar position, representing the centrists in the U.S. debate over compulsory health insurance. Like Cibrie, Delphey insisted on fee-for-service private-practice medicine and wanted to enshrine its principles in health insurance legislation. In his capacity as vice president of the Federation of Medical Economics Leagues, a New York union of doctors, Delphey opposed the AALL draft bill but accepted compulsory health insurance on principle as long as it contained "five fundamental propositions."[74] These included patient choice of physician, doctor's freedom to choose participation in an insurance fund, direct contracts between physicians and funds, and medical representation on all governing bodies. Many more physicians might have supported Delphey's initiative had they been informed of the choices before them.

The results of a survey Delphey sent to the secretaries of all state medical societies found that most of his colleagues across the country remained either uninformed or apathetic. Of the thirty-two respondents, twenty-three indicated that "the matter of Compulsory, or any other kind of Health Insurance" had never been brought before their state society and that they had no opinion whether health insurance should be entirely paid for "on the same principle that the State furnishes common school education."

None of the thirty-two state medical societies that replied to the survey had instructed its delegates to the 1916 AMA annual meeting, "either pro or con, regarding health insurance."[75] Although weak support for a centrist position undermined the cause of compulsory health insurance in the United States, it foreclosed no options concerning the course of fee-for-service private-practice medicine. Indeed, the battle over health insurance reinforced the power of U.S. practitioners nearly as much as that of their French counterparts.

Fee-for-service private-practice medicine owes much of its legitimacy not to the passage or failure of compulsory insurance but to the confrontation between state power and the individual physician's liberty of practice. Both U.S. and French doctors embraced private-practice medicine as part of doctors' struggles for professional identity and power. Although some physicians in both countries came from successful business and professional families, went to the best universities for their medical training, and could claim a high social standing in their communities, many others hailed from the lower middle class, attended medical schools of questionable reputation, and struggled to make ends meet in rural or working-class practices. For this group, compulsory health insurance might well have meant a substantial increase in income, as it had for British doctors under the National Insurance Act of 1911. In contrast to the situation in Britain, however, in the United States and France the debate over compulsory health insurance instigated a yearning among many not-so-well-off doctors for a professional identity that only an independent and entrepreneurial practice could provide.

It must be remembered that the scientific advances of the second half of the twentieth century, which propelled physicians to their present position as guardians of stupendous diagnostic technology and treatment, had not yet arrived. Many, if not most, physicians still aspired to the professional and social status of attorneys or university professors. The conflict over compulsory health insurance thus brought these aspirations to the fore and galvanized the profession as never before in a commitment to the principles of private practice and a strict adherence to charging fees for each service rendered.[76]

From this episode, then, flowed not only the AMA's extreme vigilance against subsequent initiatives for national health insurance but also the AMA's repressive efforts against its own members who pursued "nontraditional" forms of medical practice and delivery, that is, those who appeared to be departing too far from the principles that would build professional prestige and sovereignty. Although U.S. and French doctors both embraced these principles, in France the triumph of centrist physicians meant that private-practice fee-for-service medicine gained legal protections with the adoption of compulsory health insurance in 1930. Meanwhile, U.S. doctors had to rely more heavily on sheer political muscle to safeguard their professional ethics and sovereignty—muscle that eventually gave way when challenged by a vigorous managed care movement in the 1980s. Indeed, many of the conflicts over health care that bedeviled the U.S. medical profession throughout the twentieth century, including their strife over group practice beginning in the 1930s, and the waning of their control over medical decision making beginning in the 1980s, can be traced to U.S. physicians' earliest rejection of compulsory health insurance in 1918.

Divergent Fates and Futures

In April 1919, the New York State Senate, by a vote of thirty to twenty, approved the AALL's bill on compulsory health insurance, but this was the first and last legislative body to approve the measure. Due in large part to a single recalcitrant committee chairman (and manufacturer), Thaddeus Sweet, the bill never reached the New York Assembly floor. Indeed, in state after state, Progressives were repeatedly disappointed. In California, an amended AALL proposal enjoyed the support of the state's insurance commission and of Governor Hiram Johnson, who had been Theodore Roosevelt's presidential running mate on the Progressive Party's presidential ticket in 1912. In true Progressive fashion, however, the California legislature submitted the measure to voters in a referendum.

California's state medical society initially adopted a centrist approach, hoping to improve doctors' prerogatives under the law. In response, conservative physicians created the California League for the Conservation of Public Health, whose sole purpose was to defeat the referendum. On election day in November 1918, Californians trounced the measure by a margin of twenty-six percentage points, sixty-three to thirty-seven.[77] In Illinois, Pennsylvania, Wisconsin, and Massachusetts—all states that the AALL had targeted for early approval—legislative efforts failed. The early momentum of compulsory health insurance had withered in the face of public and private lobbying campaigns by insurers, physicians, employers, and their allied umbrella associations. American Federation of Labor president Samuel Gompers neutralized the support of dozens of local and state labor federations, leading critics to accuse the AALL of not really speaking for workers at all.

In 1921, AALL head John Andrews announced that the leadership had "decided to await a more favorable time before again devoting so important a part of its modest resources to [the health insurance] campaign."[78] Prominent supporters of the AALL, including the New York Federation of Labor and the Women's Joint Legislative Conference of New York, also dropped compulsory health insurance from their agendas. The United States' first battle over compulsory health insurance was over.

Meanwhile, in France, doctors fought to enshrine the freedoms of private-practice medicine in the law until the very last moment. As the legislative debate reached its height, the centrist physician Paul Cibrie founded a new professional organization, the Confédération des Syndicats Médicaux Français (CSMF), whose first task was to heal the medical profession's schism and to speak with one voice to legislators. The CSMF's first convention attracted all factions, including the conservative André Jayle and the proreformist René Lafontaine. Delegates overwhelmingly approved motions to cooperate with the government on health insurance legislation as long as the law strictly respected the principles of fee-for-service and private practice, a concession on which legislators had not yet agreed.[79]

Soon thereafter Cibrie appeared before ten thousand CGT workers, who had gathered at the Trocadero Plaza in Paris to demand that compulsory health insurance be approved with or without doctors' assent. The most powerful working-class leaders of the day brought the crowd to a fever pitch with their speeches. Unintimidated, Cibrie climbed to the podium and openly contradicted the union leaders, insisting, as he would for the next three decades, that physicians' control over medicine and medical practice must be guaranteed under any new law. Cibrie later commented: "Not since that evening have I had the opportunity to hear such a chorus of dissent, demonstrating the power of 10,000 healthy vocal cords."[80] Despite the futility of Cibrie's speech at the CGT rally, his appearance convinced any legislators who might have still doubted his resolve. Compulsory health insurance could not be achieved in France without doctors' cooperation.

The final legislation approved in April 1930 granted French physicians a "medical charter" that protected patient choice of doctor, a doctors' freedom to set fees, direct payment of medical fees, a physician's clinical freedoms, and the confidentiality of the doctor-patient relationship. For the champions of private practice, the law became a birthright. All their struggles with legislators, the acrimony among doctors, and the bitter schism of the 1920s now appeared worthwhile. The newly empowered leader of

France's now unified physicians, Paul Cibrie, called the law the "greatest victory French doctors have ever won."[81]

By all accounts, the final legislation also granted mutual leaders their demands, promising a privileged place for their organizations under the new social insurance system.[82] Indeed, one of the cosponsoring legislators labeled the emergent health insurance system "compulsory mutualism." To be sure, the government maintained powerful oversight powers, but within months of the law's implementation, the mutual movement would move to challenge the government's role even there.[83]

In the United States, the AMA celebrated the defeat of the AALL's compulsory health insurance initiative by approving a resolution that condemned "any plan embodying the system of compulsory contributory insurance against illness."[84] Such a blanket proclamation appeared to rule out the AMA's support for any kind of compulsory medical insurance. In reality, however, U.S. doctors' concerns were not so different from those of their French colleagues. U.S. physicians eventually came to be less opposed to compulsion than to the violation of private-practice freedoms and their sovereignty over medical decision making. Their ultimate enthusiasm for Medicare, which compelled workers to buy hospital insurance through wage taxes but respected physicians' freedoms, showed this beyond a doubt. Respect for private-practice medicine, however, was far from paramount among other members of the U.S. coalition that defeated compulsory health insurance after the First World War. In the absence of any consensus on the state's role in, or legal framework for, health care, U.S. employers and insurers were freer than their French counterparts to pursue their own respective goals, which inevitably brought them into conflict with doctors later in the century.

In contrast, competing interests in France had agreed to a sort of constitution under which they each fought fiercely for advantage. But the country had at least begun to construct a framework based on common ideals under which health care would be created and distributed. Despite the warnings of René Lafontaine, the emergent framework was firmly anchored to the workplace. Just as under the voluntary mutualism of the nineteenth century, an industrial worker's (now compulsory) health security remained vitally linked to employment, a trait that would last beyond the approaching Depression and war. Americans, meanwhile, would also come to embrace employment-based health insurance even more enthusiastically than the French, using it to propel the greatest expansion of health security in U.S. history, only to learn its limits in the 1970s.

3

HEALTH SECURITY, THE STATE, AND CIVIL SOCIETY, 1930–1940

We now realize as we have never realized before our interdependence on each other.

FRANKLIN DELANO ROOSEVELT, First Inaugural Address, 1933

Among large Western democracies, France and the United States were the most active social reformers in the face of the Great Depression that began in 1929. Sheer misery motivated much of this action. Reform-minded politicians, especially President Franklin Roosevelt and Prime Minister Léon Blum, enjoyed electoral successes that would have been impossible just a few years earlier. Leaders in both countries enacted social insurance and Keynesian public spending programs in an attempt to revive their stalled economies. The task in the United States was truly monumental. The gross national product of the United States plummeted 44 percent between 1929 and Roosevelt's election in 1932. The number of unemployed Americans stood at 12 million. French Depression era unemployment totaled 1.5 million, a significant figure for a country with only about a fourth the population of the United States.

In both nations, new leaders invoked images of a people united against the faceless enemy of economic crisis. Only through solidarity and joint effort, they argued, could civilization survive. For Americans, this meant unprecedented federal public works initiatives, a compulsory pension program, and national poverty assistance. In France, despite the rapidity with which the nation changed governments during the Depression—more than twenty times between 1929 and 1939—the country's powerful civil servants relentlessly pushed ahead with the implementation of compulsory health, pension, maternity, and disability insurance, which had been approved in 1930. To these laws were added major family welfare entitlements in 1932, 1938, and 1939. In 1936, the Socialist-led Popular Front government of Léon Blum granted working-class leaders a host of long-sought demands, including the ironclad protections of collective bargaining, pay hikes, and paid vacations, which enraged business and political leaders on the right.[1] After France's defeat by Nazi Germany in 1940, an authoritarian regime based in the spa town of Vichy undid much of the Popular Front's legislation benefiting workers. Independent unions were banned, as was the Confédération des Syndicats Médicaux Français (CSMF). But in its quest to remake French society, Vichy could not radically alter the basic premises of private-practice medicine that had been enshrined in the 1930 social insurance law.

In the United States, the Progressives' compulsory health insurance plan lay in tatters by 1920. By the middle of that decade, anyone who even bothered to recall the AALL's health insurance proposal would have dismissed it as an anachronism, best left to the dustbin of history. Technological innovation, nearly full employment, and vibrant economic growth seemed to have vindicated the values of individual liberty and self-help. As long as one ignored the continued disenfranchisement and poverty of African Americans and other minorities, the term "roaring" aptly captured the spirit of the 1920s. After 1920 white women could vote and, much to the chagrin of social conservatives, many insisted on driving automobiles, which were becoming ubiquitous on U.S. roadways. Anything appeared possible in the exuberance of the 1920s—cars, airplanes, art deco skyscrapers—if only government would stay out of the way. When the crash came in 1929, it was at first considered irrational; the folly that had caused it was deemed too genuinely American for blame.

Yet by 1932 the rhetoric of individual steadfastness and liberty, which promised, "Prosperity is around the corner"—President Herbert Hoover's favorite refrain—rang false in the face of a national catastrophe. Nothing could have been more different than Roosevelt's promise of a New Deal based on collective social action to spur economic recovery and to restore hope to shattered lives and the nation. Roosevelt and the Democrats took the White House and Capitol Hill by storm. A convergence of social policy in the U.S. and French republics followed. Progressive reform initiatives from the 1920s, whose European provenance was undeniable, were dusted off and served as the starting point for New Deal planning sessions.[2] Although unique to the United States, the Social Security Act of 1935 established old age insurance with benefits comparable to the French social insurance law of 1930. The American Wagner Act guaranteed workers' collective bargaining rights a year before Léon Blum's government did the same for French unions. Meanwhile, both nations created a slew of public works and poverty relief programs in hopes of priming the pumps of consumer demand.

The glaring difference between the U.S. liberals' New Deal and its *solidariste* French cousin lay in health care. In 1933, less than 6 percent of Americans had any kind of health insurance. In France, 25 percent of the population was covered under the health insurance law of 1930. By 1938, fully half of all French social insurance revenues were being spent on health care, its importance rivaled only by retirement pensions. U.S. expenditures on health care were also on the rise, but their acceleration stemmed less from government intervention than from private initiative. Because Roosevelt chose not to include health insurance in the Social Security Act of 1935 and refused to commit significant political capital to it thereafter, private actors filled the vacuum.

In the West, the industrialist Henry Kaiser was developing huge worksite group medical practices that would soon be opened to the public, a milestone that foreshadowed the transformation of U.S. health care by health maintenance organizations after 1980. Elsewhere, hospitals collaborated on prepayment plans, eventually creating a national network of hospital service plans known as Blue Cross. Not to be outdone, local medical societies created group insurance plans to pay for physician services, a development that would ultimately result in Blue Shield. All of this private initiative, however, does not mean that New Dealers in the government were inactive on the health care front. Far from it. Several of the New Deal poverty assistance programs included expansive health security programs. By far the largest was the Farm Security Administration's program to ensure medical care for the struggling rural America. By 1938 it had emerged as a nationwide program for publicly funded health care, one that trod softly and successfully around the increasingly powerful AMA, and served as a possible model for congressional action on national health insurance.

In both France and the United States, the government mediated between competing factions that sought to shape legislators' health care agenda. These factions possessed unequal resources to present their views in the halls of government power; more often than not, this inequality determined who prevailed, irrespective of the validity of their arguments. Yet all were equally subject to the reigning paradigm of fee-for-service private-practice medicine that had prevailed in the previous round of health care reform.

We must not forget that the 1930s and 1940s were also the era of Fascism, Nazism, and Stalin's consolidation of Communist power in the Soviet Union. U.S. and French proponents of private medicine were quick to identify their cause with democratic liberties and to contrast them with the menace of totalitarianism. Some physicians labeled any reform proposals that violated the sacred boundaries of private medical practice inimical to freedom. For them, the patient's choice of physician, broad clinical freedoms, the absence of third-party payers, and confidentiality between patient and doctor had become virtues as important to the survival of democracy as elections and free speech. Sadly, through innuendo and out-and-out lies, reform opponents poisoned many productive debates over the future of U.S. and French health care. This is not to say that conservatives had no right to be suspicious of reform. They were rightfully mistrustful of third parties—be they government agencies or private insurers—that sought to interfere with the doctor-patient relationship on financial grounds. Yet the conservatives' hyperbole often hindered reasoned consideration of viable solutions to the pressing problem of health insecurity.

In many ways the 1930s debate over the nature and power of health insurers has been with us ever since. Should they be government agencies, private companies, or public-private partnerships? How much authority should insurers and hospital administrators have over patient treatment? Can financial incentives to enhance productivity be designed that will not endanger the patient's best interest? How should we define health care productivity? Today, in the interest of cost savings and improved medical outcomes, U.S. and French patients willingly accept an insurer's access to knowledge that was once a closely guarded secret between patient and doctor. Our contemporary acceptance of health insurers notwithstanding, strong concerns remain in both France and the United States about medical confidentiality. The French novelist Georges Duhamel, who was also trained as a doctor, summed it up well in 1934: "The medical act is by its very essence an individual act.... It is only natural that a man, afflicted by an organic disorder, has the freedom to choose the person to whom he must confess, for good or ill, he must show himself more or less naked, feeble, wanting, miserable, or ridiculous.... The medical act is priceless.... Since the apparition of the third payer we have seen the development of a bastard industry; I call it so because it applies quantitative methods to immeasurable phenomena."[3]

In a world where purportedly rational medical science determines our pursuit of health, Duhamel portrayed the doctor as priest, the patient standing naked before God, the examining room a confessional. The Americans and the French alike embraced an idealized notion of the wise and discreet doctor whose knowledge of his patients would remain a closely guarded secret. At the same time, his increasingly impressive curative powers— aided by scientific breakthroughs—placed him on par with their minister. Thus, the charges of Communism that conservatives leveled at reformers who backed more power for third-party payers or the state were aimed not just at their politics but at their atheistic disrespect for a mythologized doctor-patient relationship. These were the tensions that lay just below the surface of many twentieth-century health care debates, occasionally rising to the surface, but always ensuring much enthusiasm and mutual incomprehension all around the table.

A New Health Care Reform Model

By 1930, advances in medical care techniques and social developments prompted the emergence of a new health care reform model. Wage replacement during illness was displaced by initiatives that emphasized payment for hospital and physician services. The appearance of this more overtly medical model stemmed in large part from the rising cost of medicine. Doctors' fees climbed steadily in the 1920s, the result of a host of overhead costs and necessary investments. Medical schools formalized their curricula, lengthening the course of study for specialists and reducing the graduation rate of others; states used medical licensing fees as a way to raise money; technological advances, including radiological and laboratory services, became an integral part of the physician's repertoire. Continuing improvements in anesthesia and antiseptics made surgeons, once disdained as butchers by physicians, into increasingly effective and sought-after specialists.

Health care inflation so outstripped wage hikes that middle-income families became concerned about their livelihoods should a medical emergency occur. Hospital beds, the vast majority of which were under government or charity purview in France and the United States, served as a safety valve for patients of limited means who needed care. But private practitioners in surrounding communities objected to losing patients to them. And it was not as if patients preferred treatment at a hospital. Interwar hospitals were only just beginning to shed their status as hostels for the indigent, mentally disturbed, tubercular, and chronically ill. Nevertheless, as everyday medical practice demanded ever-greater capital investments in operating rooms, diagnostic equipment, and laboratories, the transformation of the hospital from social prison to health care jewel gained speed.[4]

But jewels are costly. The march of modernity brought about a brutal and ironic twist. In the nineteenth century, hospitals had been repositories for sick paupers. In the twentieth, it threatened to create them. In addition to the loss of wages, those stricken by illness faced the specter of indigence resulting from the price of medical and hospital services alone, a development that demanded a change in health care reform goals. Economic and health security now meant ensuring a patient's access to sophisticated medical facilities and protection from the large medical fees for such care.

In the United States, reformers instigated a privately funded study in 1927, the Committee on the Cost on Medical Care (CCMC), to tackle the rapidly changing health care environment. In France, rising health care costs meant that reimbursement rates from the country's newly constituted compulsory health insurance funds failed to keep pace with doctors' fees, leaving patients paying far more than legislators had intended. Into the breach stepped France's mutual societies. They sought a wholesale expansion in their health care delivery capabilities as a way of holding down costs, even if they had to disregard the principles of private-practice medicine. Let us begin with the United States and the promising but ultimately contentious outcomes of the Committee on the Cost of Medical Care.

The First Search for Health Care Savings in the United States

In 1927 eight philanthropic foundations committed a million dollars to study how best to steer the development of U.S. health care.[5] At a time when such a sum was rarely available for even scientific research in medicine, the endeavor indicated a keen awareness among professional and lay observers of the vast transformation of health care that was under way. Chaired by Ray Lyman Wilbur, a physician and president of Stanford University, the committee included a mix of doctors, public health professionals, hospital administrators, insurance industry representatives, and academics. Generous funding permitted a full-time staff of seventy-five statisticians and technical experts, many of whom would go on to play significant roles in New Deal and postwar health care initiatives. The committee staff fanned out across the country, producing over two dozen field reports on various approaches to health care in rural and urban settings. Their examination of previously little-known community and employer health care efforts had a profound effect on reform initiatives for the next twenty years, especially in the areas of prepayment and group practice, where they documented substantial equity, cost, and access improvements.

One of the most illuminating was an employer-sponsored plan in Roanoke Rapids, North Carolina. There five textile and paper mill employers had built a single medical complex that included a hospital, diagnostic services (X-rays and laboratories), and the offices of community physicians. Physicians received above-average salaries for the care of mill workers and were free to receive at the clinic patients unassociated with the mills. The entire operation was financed through a group prepayment plan under which workers paid approximately one-third and employers two-thirds of total outlays.[6] Findings of the study unequivocally favored group practice. Mill workers obtained more medical care for less money than their non–mill worker neighbors, comparing favorably with those with incomes over ten thousand dollars—a substantial annual income for the period. The quality of medicine was also rated high; and the burden of medical costs was generalized to the entire mill-working population instead of being restricted to an unlucky few. As strong as its findings were, the CCMC report on Roanoke's group practice contained blind spots that would bedevil U.S. health care reformers for decades.

CCMC researchers ignored race. African Americans constituted only 16 percent of the township population but a majority in the surrounding county, which also depended on the medical center. Blacks used the hospital far less than white non–mill workers, presumably because of their lower incomes but also because of racial discrimination. Blacks were treated only after all whites had been seen; they also had to enter by a separate door and use a separate waiting room. The CCMC recognized the deplorable conditions of African American health and health care services but explained them away as "not surprising." This attitude was not unusual for the day, but it undermined researchers' larger conclusions concerning the viability of the Roanoke Rapids medical center.[7]

In their overall assessment of the group practice, researchers perceptively noted that the hospital and associated ambulatory care center would provide residents with more health security if it were funded through a communitywide tax. As it turned out, when the Depression hit, mill owners did cut back on health care funding, thereby demonstrating the precarious nature of employer-reliant programs. Yet for all their foresight, CCMC researchers were blind to the fact that the dominant African American population in the county would be unlikely to agree to pay taxes for a facility that perpetuated an oppressive and medically dangerous racism.[8] African Americans' access to health care facilities in southern states would become a major point of contention between reformers and Southern congressional representatives in the 1960s. In the meantime, the CCMC's research, which pointed to the advantages of group practice and prepayment, opened an unbridgeable rift between committee members.

Committee members so disagreed on how to interpret the findings of staff research that separate majority and minority reports had to be filed. The majority of the CCMC (thirty-nine of fifty members) sided with staff findings concerning the desirability of group practice and health insurance. They concluded that "medical services, both preventative and therapeutic, should be furnished largely by organized groups of physicians, dentists, nurses, pharmacists, and other associated personnel."[9] The majority based its recommendation on evidence from Roanoke Rapids and elsewhere showing that the growing necessity of capital investments, coupled with a trend toward medical specialization, as well as traditional overhead costs—rent, supplies, office space—made group practice more efficient and therefore more economical for patients and doctors alike. The majority believed that patients could exercise sufficient choice of physician and build meaningful doctor-patient relationships within the constraints of group practice.

The majority of the CCMC also left no doubt that they considered health care an arena where the principles of equality and risk sharing should trump individual liberty and self-help. Indeed, several members of the majority openly favored compulsory health insurance. They noted that "no legerdemain can bring into a voluntary [health insurance] system the unorganized, low-paid working group who are not indigent but live on a minimum subsistence income." They also predicted that "vested interests are built up under voluntary insurance which are very difficult to dislodge, even though they seriously hamper effective work."[10]

The minority would have none of it. Physicians made up eight of the nine dissenters who prepared the minority report. (Two other members filed reports separate from both the majority and the minority.) They objected that the majority's recommendation of group practice flew in the face of the committee's agreed-on premise to protect the personal doctor-patient relationship. In language that recalls that of the Frenchman Georges Duhamel, though less poetic, the minority report insisted that by "personal relationship is meant that bond of sympathy . . . and mutual regard for each other which cause the patient to disclose for purpose of diagnosis and treatment the most private and confidential information concerning himself . . . intimacy . . . that assumes priestly characteristics on the part of the physician."[11] In the absence of such a relationship, charged the dissenters, "mass" practice would debase the quality of medicine and its practitioners. They argued instead that, while group practices may make sense in a limited number of communities where all practitioners could be grouped into one or two facilities, in most areas of the country group practices would not only destroy the doctor-patient relationship, they would lead to excess capital investment and abet what they viewed as a troubling trend toward specialization of practice: "It serves no good purpose to reduce overhead in individual clinics if the total cost to the community is increased through the duplication of plants."[12]

The physicians of the CCMC minority assumed a doctrinaire position quite similar to that taken by Paul Cibrie, the triumphant leader of France's doctors. Cibrie had accepted insurance—in his case compulsory insurance—but only if it bolstered physician sovereignty under fee-for-service private-practice medicine. U.S. and French doctors abhorred "contract practices," which the AMA's Judicial Council defined as the furnishing of services "to a group or class of individuals for a definite sum or for a fixed rate per capita." Such arrangements occurred when doctors offered care to a fraternal order or to workers of an entire industrial plant. It constituted a blatant violation of private fee-for-service medicine and evoked the punitive wrath of U.S. and French medical leaders. Just as French doctors had done only a few years before, the CCMC minority insisted that what mattered most was not *whether* to accept or block health insurance but rather *who* administers and *who* controls the insurer. The minority accepted the possibility of insurance but only if it were controlled by physicians acting through a local medical society and with nonprofit status. Only with these safeguards in place, they believed, would the sanctity of private medicine be secure.[13]

When all was said and done, the physicians who wrote the minority report proved far more influential in determining the direction of U.S. health care than the majority. Their careful acceptance of health insurance blazed a trail that would be trod by countless AMA officials and their political supporters for the next fifty years. The minority report also opened the way for physician support of early hospital prepayment plans, which would evolve into Blue Cross and the medical profession's own foray into health insurance, Blue Shield.

French Mutual Aid Societies and Managed Care

The growing complexity of health care and its attendant costs in the 1930s fueled a comparable struggle over the cost and nature of private medicine in France, albeit within the framework of compulsory health insurance. Like their U.S. counterparts, French doctors had committed themselves to protect private medicine and had tied their professional status to spreading it. Yet no sooner had the law been approved than the country's preeminent insurers, the mutual aid societies, indicated that they viewed fee-for-service medicine as a luxury. It was all well and good for those who could afford it, but it should not restrict the development of other forms of health care provision. As in the U.S. debate at the CCMC, group practice and the doctor-patient relationship played central roles in their reasoning.

Under France's 1930 health insurance legislation, a social insuree who sought medical care enjoyed free choice of physician.[14] He was required to pay his doctor's bill in full, based on a fee schedule that had been negotiated between his health insurance fund and the local medical *syndicat*. The patient then sought reimbursement, 80 percent for most procedures, from the fund. In practice, however, relations between mutual societies, which administered many health insurance funds, and doctors' *syndicats* quickly became strained over fees. In effect, physicians came to view the fee schedules as minimum charges rather than, as had been intended by legislators, delimited maximums. What is more, since the revenues came from legally defined wage and payroll taxes, mutual societies could not raise insurance premiums to match physician fee hikes. Caught in the middle, of course, were patients, who often found themselves with doctors' bills that their health insurance would reimburse at the rate of only 40 or 50 percent.[15]

Doctors insisted that they should be free to practice medicine with the sole interest of the patient in mind, irrespective of cost considerations. Mutual societies, conversely, accused doctors of using the presence of a third-party payer to raise prices, in some cases in violation of the contracts that their *syndicats* had signed. But in fact, an individual doctor was not legally bound by any contract between his medical *syndicat* and the local health insurance fund—the individual liberty of the physician under private medicine prohibited it.[16] In response, mutual societies cast themselves in the role of savior and sought to provide medical services to patients at lower prices; but in so doing, they violated the most sacrosanct principles of private medicine.

If French doctors had obtained legal protections for private practice under France's compulsory health insurance law, then how could the mutual movement possibly pose a danger to doctors? The answer lay in a contradiction. Although the law expressly sanctioned private practice, it also granted mutual aid societies the right to use their existing medical infrastructure to "benefit their members who are insurees under the present law."[17] In 1930 mutual societies were far from able to offer complete medical services; they typically only owned pharmacies and small dispensaries for the convenience of their members.

As implementation of the law proceeded, mutual leaders realized that their role as insurance carriers put them on the receiving end of an endless barrage of patient complaints about insufficient reimbursement for independent practitioners' medical services. Without more control over prices, they would soon become nothing but unpopular agents of a government-directed health insurance bureaucracy. Mutual leaders reckoned the only way to stem their slide into oblivion would be to stretch the law's loophole regarding mutual health care facilities to seize control of prices, that is, to become health care providers in their own right.

According to this vision, a patient should be able to choose between a fee-for-service practitioner and comparable medical services provided by a mutual society. The success of the initiative would be assured if mutual societies could provide quality services that eliminated the yawning gap between doctors' fees and health insurance reimbursement. The mutual movement certainly enjoyed fantastic exposure to the target population. They administered 80 percent of local health insurance funds; they also had many middle-class subscribers who were not subject to compulsory health insurance but would nonetheless seek care at new facilities, especially as the efficacy and price of medical care continued to rise.[18] Propelled by this rationale, the mutual movement aggressively moved to acquire health care plants and equipment.[19] Mutual societies banded together into regional unions, pooling sufficient funds to build surgery and diagnostic centers across France.

These facilities presented a conundrum for physicians. By doctrine they had to condemn the subordinate contract positions that surgeons assumed in the mutual society surgery centers. They also deplored the fact that patients had little choice of their surgeon and that payment for medical services was handled through the mutual society, not directly between the patient and medical practitioner. Worse still, it soon became apparent that many surgeons liked to practice under such circumstances. The mutual centers often possessed the latest available technology and offered rewarding contracts or regular salaries. Even more nettlesome, surgeons who practiced in the mutual society–run centers typically paid generous referral fees to community physicians. By 1939 there were six surgery insurance funds run by mutual societies, with nearly a million subscribers. The sheer financial power of the mutual movement made it a formidable opponent of the medical profession. In the northern department of Pas de Calais, mutual societies simply purchased two of the four existing surgery facilities and promptly contracted with five local surgeons, who then substantially undercut customary local surgical fees. In this way, the mutual movement's deep pockets permitted it to successfully compete with private fee-for-service medicine.[20]

Mutual society laboratories and X-ray centers also presented a threat to private practitioners because they were usually paired with group medical practices nearby. Aided by their access to labs and imaging centers, the group practices not only successfully competed with private-practice doctors, they also preached a new approach to care that emphasized prevention over curative medicine. A 1944 survey revealed 139 mutual health clinics nationwide, many of them specializing in maternal and well-baby care, and general physical fitness. The same survey indicated that mutual societies controlled twenty dental offices and forty-two pharmacies.[21]

Yet no matter how much mutual doctors advocated health maintenance, it was the move into curative care on the part of mutual societies that piqued France's medical leaders. With this care, together with the surgery centers, the mutual movement was well on its way to building a parallel health care delivery system that could displace private-practice physicians who adhered to fee-for-service medicine. As one mutual leader put it in 1933, "The wish of mutual societies is to create everywhere feasible, even in the smallest towns... comprehensive general medical services. First will be dispensaries, true centers of prevention.... Next will come convalescence and curative facilities, such as sanatoria and hospitals."[22] If the mutual movement had its way, doctors on contract or receiving salaries would provide medical services at all these facilities.

France's medical profession fought back with a vengeance.[23] Physicians sought and finally obtained some practice privileges in public hospitals so that private-practice physicians could treat patients there. Previously, only the indigent were admitted to public hospitals, and salaried government physicians provided nearly all treatment. Yet even after this breakthrough, private practitioners remained at a disadvantage. Public hospitals remained part and parcel of France's system of poverty relief. They hardly resembled the comprehensive health care centers that were being built by mutual aid societies, facilities that truly prefigured the gleaming complexes of late-century French medical care.

Medical association leader Paul Cibrie openly urged local medical *syndicats* to respond to the mutual movements in kind. Local *syndicats*,

Cibrie suggested, should create "regional medical centers that are extensions of physician offices...to provide expensive technologies that the doctor cannot by himself afford."[24] Thus French doctors banded together to build their own modern surgery centers and diagnostic clinics, sometimes with the financial support of local employers. Cibrie rallied doctors with rhetoric that portrayed the mutual movement as an invading totalitarian army. "In the face of a lightning offensive launched by the mutual movement's general staff...all doctors are reminded of the principles of [private medicine]....We want French medicine to remain as it is, to guard its freedoms, and to become in our own time one of the most unyielding champions of individual liberty."[25] Of most concern to medical leaders was the mutual movement's legislative attack on the legal safeguards of fee-for-service medicine that doctors had won in their compromise on compulsory health insurance.

In 1933 mutual society allies in Parliament sponsored a bill that would have explicitly permitted societies to channel social insurees to specific practitioners. If approved, private practitioners would likely have found it necessary to sign contracts to deliver care with local mutual society provider networks. Under these circumstances, without legal protection, private-practice medicine would have been vulnerable to cost-efficiency calculations in the face of a massive consolidation in medical services. As Cibrie warned his colleagues, "If we don't win this fight [against the mutual society bill]...in one year we'll all be working for mutual societies, not as state doctors, in which case we'd have a pension, but as workers; we'll have nothing."[26]

The mutual movement's legislative offensive against fee-for-service medicine, however, proved an overreach. It so enraged physicians that they unholstered their ultimate weapon. In a remarkable display of professional solidarity, France's physicians threatened that, if the bill were to become law, "the French medical profession, in its entirety, would immediately cease its collaboration with the [health insurance] law."[27] In light of the discipline that physicians had demonstrated to gain legal protections for private medicine in 1930, few believed that the doctors were bluffing. More important, however, no political leader wished to challenge openly the still-popular values of patient choice, physician's clinical freedoms, and medical confidentiality. Public opinion of the health insurance law was low enough as it was. The will to change it, even to deliver on grand promises of more affordable care, faltered before the fear of losing individualized medicine, to which French workers had grown accustomed. The failure of the mutual society–sponsored bill not only resulted in a further strengthening of fee-for-service medicine, it also channeled the mutual movement's expansion energies toward middle-class patients who were not yet covered by compulsory health insurance.[28]

Union leaders had watched the conflict between mutual societies and doctors with great interest. They were intrigued by the direction that mutual leaders wished to take French health care. But in the 1930s they would go no further than a philosophical statement about the need "to move away from traditional, purely individual and curative medicine, and toward social medicine, which is preventative and defensive, an evolution that is imperative for the public health of the country."[29] When it came to concrete proposals, labor leaders demurred, preferring to give the new law more time. They also put off improving their relations with doctors, which the unions admitted were "far from perfect."[30]

The attitude of France's labor leaders, together with the mutual movement's aborted attack on fee-for-service medicine, demonstrate that France's historic health care compromise was holding. To be sure, local skirmishes over mutual society—run clinics and their salaried doctors continued, but at the national level the 1930 health insurance law was a success. It embraced a sufficient measure of collective equality by compelling employers and workers to share the cost of health care across a broad segment of the population, about 25 percent, or nearly 10 million people, by 1940. Simultaneously, legislators had held fast to personal liberty by sanctioning the individualism intrinsic to private-practice medicine. This dual approach permitted a nation that had been firmly attached to voluntary health security solutions to reconcile liberty with equality. Mutual societies played an indispensable role in this transition by serving as a trusted intermediary between the government and the individual. Government intervention existed in law, but for many workers it came clothed in the familiar dress of their local mutual society. When mutual leaders sought legislative approval for a further collectivization of French medicine, they ran into a wall of opposition from doctors and a decided lack of enthusiasm from union leaders, lawmakers, and the general public. Workers were understandably upset with the disappointing reimbursements for medical services, yet these same workers fervently believed in patient choice, physician's liberty of medical practice, and the sanctity of the doctor-patient relationship.

A strict maintenance of medical confidentiality laws was integral to the compromise that opened the way for compulsory health insurance in France. That law is essentially unchanged today: physicians who revealed "secrets confided in them by their patients, unless compelled by a legal authority which may oblige their disclosure" could be imprisoned for up to six months and were subject to substantial fines, not to mention revocation of their medical license.[31]

At first blush, the medical confidentiality law looks like a mere detail in the evolution of twentieth-century health care. Nothing could be further from the truth. Medical secrecy serves as an important marker of the strength of private-practice medicine as health insurance is gaining strength, for it mirrors the professional secrecy and discipline that doctors demand of one another vis-à-vis the state and society. When a physician speaks of his special knowledge after "he has plunged his scrutinizing eye under the hidden-most folds of [his patient's] soul," that physician cannot help but feel entitled to extend his prerogatives beyond the doctor-patient relationship to the larger field of medicine, its organization, and its relationship with society.[32] The increasing efficacy of medicine, coupled with more rigorous clinical training, permitted physicians to claim more and more sovereignty over health care affairs. Private-practice medicine became both a creed for professional sovereignty and the basis for its protection. At its center lay the private doctor-patient relationship. From there, the other principles—freedom of diagnosis and therapy, patient choice of physician, and fee-for-service—were arrayed like defensive fortifications to protect notions of quality medicine as defined by doctors themselves.

Because of the compromise they reached on compulsory health insurance in 1930, French doctors never pushed the boundaries of professional sovereignty as far as their U.S. counterparts. But by century's end, when the medical profession in both countries was fighting rearguard actions to protect its prerogatives over medical decision making, French physicians succeeded far more effectively in protecting the innermost sanctums of private practice.[33]

In the 1930s, however, U.S. doctors were still hard at work building their professional sovereignty. One of their most able spokesmen was Morris Fishbein, editor of the *Journal of the American Medical Association*. He insisted that "no other group except physicians is really entitled to say how medicine shall be practiced, for only the physicians are competent...to judge adequately the quality of medical care. There is no criterion of adequate medical care except the quality of the care that is rendered." Fishbein's argument was, of course, syllogistic and therefore impossible to disprove, unless laypeople could examine and question the evidence concerning the quality of care. What is more, Fishbein maintained that it was "useless to attempt to distinguish between the content of medical practice and the method of administration."[34]

Thus, according to Fishbein, all of the most important issues concerning the new model for health care—compulsory versus voluntary health insurance, group practice, prepayment for hospital care, and the proper administrator for any new entities that reforms might create—could not be decided without the explicit consent of the AMA. Without a doubt, Fishbein's expansive view of the medical profession's sovereignty reflected the AMA's anxiety about President Roosevelt's plans to include compulsory health insurance in the New Deal.

The New Deal and Health Care

The 1932 presidential contest between the Democrat Franklin Roosevelt and the Republican incumbent Herbert Hoover turned on the candidates' different remedies for the Depression and social reform; health care per se was not a campaign issue. The Democratic platform pledged federal aid for the rural areas and support for veterans' pensions, but it also promised a reduction in federal spending and a balanced budget. Systematic health care reform along the lines recommended by the CCMC majority was nowhere to be seen. Nonetheless, a general anxiety spread in Republican circles about the contours of Roosevelt's promised "New Deal," exacerbated by a lame-duck period that at the time stretched from November until March. Indeed, Hoover openly asked for assurances from the president-elect that he was not contemplating any radical measures, a request that Hoover felt necessary to calm a winter banking crisis. The deft Roosevelt responded reassuringly without making any assurances.

In this context, an editorial in the *Journal of the American Medical Association (JAMA)* came as a preemptive volley directed at possible New Deal health care initiatives. The editors pronounced that the "alignment is clear—on the one side the forces representing the great foundations, public health officials and social theory—even socialism and communism—inciting to revolution; on the other side, the organized medical profession of this country urging an orderly evaluation guided by controlled experimentation which will observe principles that have been found through the centuries to be necessary to the sound practice of medicine."[35] The AMA's attempt to associate health care reformers with Communist revolutionaries was hardly the first or last of its kind.

Many opponents of the New Deal considered it un-American, and health care reformers in particular were subjected to a fierce barrage of ad hominem attacks throughout the 1930s and 1940s.[36] If the Committee on the Cost of Medical Care's recommendations had already set members of the AMA on edge, Roosevelt's early leadership appointments made them even more anxious. The president chose a reform-minded Wisconsin professor, Edwin Witte, to head the newly created Committee on Economic Security (CES). Edgar Sydenstricker, a well-known proponent of compulsory health insurance, was charged with the CES's Technical Committee on Medical Care. I. S. Falk, another health care reformer from the CCMC, became Sydenstricker's chief staff assistant and brought several like-minded CCMC researchers with him. Still more worrisome for reform opponents was the plight of their own camp.

Commercial insurers, who had funded an array of umbrella organizations to counter the earlier compulsory health insurance initiative, had been debilitated by the Depression. Virtually all of them were either in or near bankruptcy, forcing their leaders to call upon Roosevelt hat in hand. Roosevelt duly obliged them, authorizing loans backed by the Reconstruction Finance Corporation of the federal government. Once on the public dole, however, the previously powerful commercial insurance lobby could do little more than whisper their alarm at the growing strength of health care reform forces.

Fraternal orders, which had played a critical grassroots role in the insurance industry's fight against the earlier health insurance bill, were similarly hamstrung by the economic crisis. Many of their leaders looked to Roosevelt to save them from insolvency, caused by mass unemployment and homelessness. Indeed, only through extraordinary public measures did many fraternal orders survive the Depression. The government's massive inroads into poverty relief and social insurance relieved struggling societies of their most burdensome members. Fraternal members were hardly inclined to participate in a letter-writing campaign against Roosevelt, who offered them relief in trying times. Consequently, most fraternal leaders gave their implied consent, if not outspoken support, for the New Deal.[37]

Organized labor's position had also changed. In the previous battle over compulsory health insurance, AFL leader Samuel Gompers had bitterly opposed government intervention, arguing instead that workers' unions ought to seek independent solutions based on individual choice and liberty. William Green, however, who had taken over the reins of the AFL in 1924, adopted the opposite position. Green had been a founding member of the United Mine Workers of America, where he represented workers particularly vulnerable to ill health and injury. In recognition of labor's importance to the New Deal coalition and Green's support for social insurance, Roosevelt appointed him to the CES, where he strenuously argued for the inclusion of health insurance in the definition of economic security. Thus, the coalition that had defeated compulsory health insurance in 1920 had been whittled down to the AMA and employers. And even these well-respected lobbies appeared vulnerable in the tumult of the Depression.

In his 1933 inaugural address, Roosevelt spoke at length about the financial crisis afflicting the nation, hardly a surprising choice since so many Americans had lost their life savings in bank failures. But Roosevelt went well beyond promises to restore a crippled banking system. He scornfully attacked bankers for their "false leadership" and pledged to "apply social values" in restoring the country's banks. A major portion of the new president's speech was devoted to an attack on the professional sovereignty of bankers, members of a hallowed U.S. profession, and argued for massive government intrusion in banking practices. This appeal, side by side with Roosevelt's repeated recognition of the citizenry's "interdependence on each other . . . we can not merely take but we must give as well,"[38] led AMA leaders to assume that the president regarded doctors' sovereignty not as inalterable but as contingent on the social needs of the nation. Given the unmet medical needs of the population, many AMA officials further assumed that Roosevelt was preparing a new health insurance offensive.

But the attack never came. The administration made only a few tentative thrusts to gauge the AMA's strength and to ascertain the damage that doctors could inflict on the larger New Deal project. While Sydenstricker and Falk enthusiastically planned to include health insurance in the Social Security Act, Labor Secretary Frances Perkins and CES Director Witte grew increasingly concerned about a melee over health care. The White House had been receiving a steady stream of letters and telegrams from doctors who opposed any New Deal initiatives on medical care, the product of a nationwide medical society campaign orchestrated by the AMA. Newspaper editorials also began to appear, making the same arguments as the doctors' letters. Despite the public campaign that had begun against them, Sydenstricker and Falk insisted that a large portion of the medical profession would eventually support compulsory health insurance, just as many British practitioners had belatedly embraced the National Insurance Act of 1911.

Sydenstricker and Falk believed that once medical leaders had been invited to sit on a Medical Advisory Committee, the opposition would subside and give way to political bargaining over the shape of legislation. But throughout the fall of 1934, the letters kept coming. Sydenstricker sought to reassure Witte. He emphasized that several prominent medical leaders had agreed to participate in the government's Medical Advisory Committee even as the AMA's public opposition continued. For Sydenstricker, this meant deep divisions within the medical profession, a circumstance that the administration could use to its advantage. In November 1934, however, when physicians who they had believed were either neutral or mildly proreform broadsided Sydenstricker and Falk at their own roundtable, Witte had had enough. He and Perkins advised Roosevelt to drop health insurance from the Social Security Act for fear it would jeopardize the entire bill. The sagacity of this advice became apparent during the House Ways and Means Committee hearings. Such a chorus of lawmakers spoke against health insurance that a majority of the committee insisted that even its mention as a topic of research be struck from the act.[39]

Roosevelt could only have been impressed by the AMA's show of force and the concomitant weakness of pro–health insurance groups. The AFL, the CIO, and farm bureaus failed to rally anywhere near a comparable display of congressional support. Health insurance, in contrast to old age pensions and unemployment insurance, appeared to have lost the reform energy it had enjoyed in the days of the AALL campaign between 1916 and 1920.[40] Heeding this message, Roosevelt suppressed a favorable CES report on health insurance for fear it would hurt his chances in the 1936 elections. Although Roosevelt never publicly conceded defeat on compulsory health insurance, he never again risked substantial political capital to achieve it.

The seemingly gratuitous action by the House Ways and Means Committee offered a glimpse of the dilemma faced by Roosevelt and every one of his successors, through Bill Clinton. It also demonstrated how race once again entered the equation of health care security. Southern Democrats had benefited disproportionately from Roosevelt's 1932 Democratic landslide, and their leaders continued their ascension to the chairs of a congressional committee system that rewarded seniority. Despite the unquestioned urgency of New Deal relief, the Democratic Party's southern wing was troubled by Roosevelt's massive expansion of federal executive power—power that Republican and Democratic conservatives alike viewed as a danger to states' rights. If the president pushed his Southern Democratic colleagues too hard, he risked mass defections, which could have brought the New Deal and Roosevelt's own continued electoral success to a halt.[41]

Thus, the AMA's campaign against compulsory health insurance, impressive in and of itself, also fell on very fertile ground. The AMA was a confederation and therefore quite capable of cultivating regional leaders who could lobby their members of Congress in the local dialect. Their insistence that government-sponsored health insurance constituted a massive federal invasion targeting medical sovereignty and would crush the traditions of private-practice medicine served as a poignant metaphor for Southerners' bitter history with federal power. Unlike compulsory health insurance, the Social Security Act's headline features—old age and unemployment insurance—were not comparably invasive. Both employers and workers were asked to contribute on equal terms to a pension system that remained firmly linked to private labor markets, and business leaders supported it.[42]

Even then, southern legislators obtained the exclusion of agricultural and domestic labor from participation in Social Security and a host of New Deal relief programs, including National Recovery, Agricultural Adjustment, National Labor Relations, and the Fair Labor Standards Acts, thereby depriving 90 percent of the southern African American workforce from most New Deal benefits. As the historian Colin Gordon explains, the "implications of the agricultural exclusion were also quite clearly specific to the South and Southwest—regions whose economies were dominated by agriculture, whose agricultural systems were peculiarly labor intensive, and whose agricultural labor markets were organized around low wages, tenancy, harsh legal controls, and violence."[43] Once reformers moved from a state-by-state strategy, which had focused on the North and Midwest, to a national health insurance big bang, southern lawmakers emerged as a stumbling block. After Roosevelt was reelected in 1936, reformers inside and outside his administration had little choice but to try to build more public support for health security measures, an effort that led them to sponsor a National Health Conference in Washington.

The conference opened on 18 July 1938 at Washington's Mayflower Hotel. One hundred and fifty delegates represented the broadest array of heath care interests that had ever been assembled at a single gathering. As the conference wore on, consensus emerged on a variety of issues, including hospital construction, the expansion of maternal and child health, and initiatives to meet the medical needs of the indigent. But conferees diverged sharply when they considered proposals to create "a comprehensive program designed to increase and improve medical services for the entire population," to be funded by taxes or insurance premiums. The administration's I. S. Falk rose to defend an insurance proposal, delivering an impassioned speech that made every possible argument in favor of compulsory health insurance: it would alleviate medical indigence; distribute the burden of health care costs; create economies of scale in medical plant and equipment; promote the virtues of contributory social insurance while preserving individual dignity; and leave wide latitude to states and localities for implementation.[44] Although conferees had agreed in advance that no formal vote on their National Health Program would be conducted, support for health insurance ran wide and deep among participants.

The AMA moved swiftly to combat this second wave of New Deal health care activism launched by the National Health Conference. The editor of *JAMA,* Fishbein, launched an extensive publicity campaign, again aimed at members of Congress, insisting that compulsory health insurance constituted "another step towards the breakdown of American democracy and a trend toward a system fascistic or communistic in character directly opposed to the democratic principle."[45] In 1939 Senator Robert Wagner of New York braved the AMA and introduced legislation to enact the National Health Conference program, including state-run programs for compulsory health insurance. Indeed, much as Medicaid does today, the Wagner bill would have provided the states great leeway on how to construct their health insurance programs. This, it was hoped, might engender a modicum of support from conservative Southern Democratic legislators, who would appreciate the concession to states' rights. But Wagner's bill went nowhere. Despite the Democratic majority, conservative Southerners in key leadership positions refused to provide needed support.

Roosevelt's early flirtation with health insurance as part of the Social Security Act, followed by reformers' vigorous manifestation at the National Health Conference, emboldened diverse players already on the field. By far the keenest observers of the New Deal's inaction on health security were the fledgling Blue Cross hospital service plans and proponents of group medical practices. Employers too were quick to learn the lessons of the New Deal's failure to enact health insurance. They were now free to create health care benefits for their workers without fear of seeing those programs made superfluous by federal mandates. The industrialist Henry Kaiser, whose prosperity resulted from the New Deal's western public works programs, expanded his group health care on such a scale that he earned the condemnation of the AMA. Others such as Kodak, Sears, and Thompson dutifully respected physicians' professional sovereignty and private medicine while building "modern manors" that portended a new generation of welfare capitalist employers.[46]

In a way, the Blues and employers benefited twice over from the brouhaha over compulsory health insurance. In the first place, they profited from a national debate about inadequate health security that frightened the public but did nothing to allay that danger. Second, as invincible as the AMA appeared, even the most conservative medical leaders realized that intransigence in the face of reformers could not prevail forever. The AMA would need to make a strategic shift toward prepayment for hospital services and group medical care insurance if the profession wished to remain in control. Hence, not only did the impasse of compulsory health insurance under the New Deal create a vacuum into which nonstate actors could step, the very nature of its failure, resulting from the appeal to the principles of private medicine and professional sovereignty, further propelled a divergence between French and U.S. health care.

French doctors successfully relied on the social insurance law of 1930 to stem the incursion of mutual societies into health care delivery and to prop up private-practice medicine. In the absence of any national health care policy, the AMA built a far more extensive and robust political organization than did French doctors. U.S. medical leaders not only had to combat insurgencies from a more diverse set of actors, including some within their own ranks, they also needed to demonstrate the profession's ability to lead constructive reform during an unprecedented transformation in medical services.

Civil Society Organizations and the Birth of Blue Cross and Blue Shield

Civil society organizations are voluntary groups that operate independently of traditional market pressures and state power. In the social arena, they often serve an intermediary role between the government and citizens. In the realm of health security, many groups could rightfully claim the title of civil society organization in the 1930s. Faith-based charities, voluntary hospitals, and fraternal orders topped the list. Mutual aid societies constituted France's premier health care civil society organizations. Their widespread popularity and nongovernmental status enabled them to play a crucial advocacy role in the passage of the country's 1930 health insurance law. Thereafter, mutual societies became a pivotal administrative intermediary in implementing the law. The French mutual movement made compulsory health insurance palatable to a society that had long preferred voluntary associations and individual self-help as the path to health security.

One might suppose that fraternal orders were the comparable institution in the United States. Certainly, in terms of historical origins and legal status, the comparison is plausible. French mutual societies and U.S. fraternal orders both constituted essential elements of nineteenth-century social welfare in their respective countries. Both attracted members who shared ethnic affinities or socioeconomic status—usually working-class and petty bourgeois men who wished to protect themselves from the risks of illness, accident, and old age. Many mutual societies and fraternal orders also enjoyed privileged relationships with local philanthropic groups, charities, and employers. Both also constructed a social welfare infrastructure, including health care facilities. Yet, lengthy as this list of commonalities may be, U.S. fraternal orders and French mutual societies diverged abruptly in the 1920s.

In contrast to its French counterpart, the U.S. fraternal movement opposed efforts to pass compulsory health insurance in the United States. Shortly after doing so, the fraternal movement suffered a series of devastating blows. Strict postwar immigration restrictions, aimed particularly at southern and eastern Europe, slowed membership growth to a trickle, prompting an erosion of political and financial standing. Then, after 1929, the Depression decimated fraternals' already ailing financial reserves. Finally, income tax policies made group insurance premiums tax deductible but left individual payments, commonly used by fraternal orders, fully taxable.[47]

The tax deductibility of group insurance premiums marked the first of many tax policies whose effect on twentieth-century U.S. health care cannot be overemphasized. It created a windfall advantage to organizations that sold group health policies and further undermined the already-weak fraternals. Commercial insurers and civil society organizations that cracked the group insurance market thrived in the 1930s and beyond. Foremost among these were Blue Cross hospital plans, which during their formative years exhibited many of the same traits, including tensions with doctors, as France's mutual aid societies.

The Depression spelled deep trouble for U.S. hospitals. Per capita receipts had fallen an amazing 74 percent. Hospital deficits rose, while occupancy rates plummeted. Community and private hospital board members across the country were frantic to avoid closing their doors for lack of financial resources—"just 30 days ahead of the sheriff," as one of them put it. The answer to hospitals' woes came from Texas, where an enterprising Baylor University administrator, Justin Ford Kimball, had been hired to shore up the sagging finances of the university's hospital. Kimball conceived group hospital prepayment plans when a young middle manager, Bryce Twitty, asked him why they "couldn't do for sick people what lumber camps and railroads had done for their employees."[48]

Within weeks, Kimball was in contract negotiations with the Dallas school district, where he had once served as superintendent, to provide teachers with a way to budget against future hospital expenses. In exchange for fifty cents a month from each teacher, Baylor University offered twenty-one days of hospital care per year, meals, nursing, and professional staff care, including operating room and laboratory services, anesthesia, medications, dressings, and casts. By 1934, Kimball and Twitty had signed up 408 area employers—23,000 employees in all. Although Kimball and Twitty's initiative translated into a welcome surge of hospital revenue, it also constituted an unprecedented liability for Baylor. Fully aware of the danger, Kimball looked in vain for actuarial data that might help him manage his brainchild.[49]

It was not as if Kimball was a rookie. He had worked as an insurance lawyer and therefore knew where the largest financial danger lay: moral hazard. To avoid moral hazard, the liabilities that are insured against must be both unambiguous when they occur and beyond the control of the insured. If they are not, the insurer cannot accurately predict costs, and the presence of insurance itself may increase claims and therefore losses.[50] Moral hazard avoidance measures dictate that insurers carefully control their issuance of individual policies to guard against, for example, the presence of preexisting medical conditions. Kimball was not selling insurance but rather hospital benefits, but the problem of moral hazard remained.

Baylor provided hospital services directly to members in exchange for their premiums; there was no cash indemnity or third party. The hospital was fully liable but also fully in control, theoretically anyway, of the costs of its own services. However important this difference, it could not entirely attenuate the problem of moral hazard. What did, however, was employee group payment. Kimball's epiphany had come when he was asked about paternalistic industrialists' management of health care for their workers. By definition, members of employee groups possessed a reasonable level of health; otherwise, they would be incapable of remaining employed. If an individual fell too ill, became too old, or suffered too serious an accident to keep working, then he or she, again by definition, lost membership in the group prepayment plan and ceased to exist as a source of service claims and losses for the hospital. Such exclusions were exactly what had troubled the

French medical leader René Lafontaine about employer-physician alliances just a few years before.

A second method of guarding against moral hazard concerned the group itself. Baylor Hospital's contract with Dallas schools stipulated that at least 75 percent of teachers subscribe to the plan. This not only assured the hospital a minimum revenue, it also diluted the plan's losses from moral hazard, that is to say, from members whose reason for seeking hospital admittance existed prior to eligibility or was ambiguous in origin. To further safeguard the solvency of the plan, Kimball precluded any treatment for chronic afflictions, including pulmonary tuberculosis, mental illness, nervous system disorders, and smallpox. Plan benefits also excluded treatment for venereal diseases; the moral stigma attached to them undoubtedly assured that no objections would be raised. Maternity care, a potentially expensive service, was covered at the rate of only 50 percent. Kimball and Twitty's deft judgments on price and utilization, in the absence of actuarial data, resulted in a landmark success for Baylor University Hospital and the creation of a replicable model for hospital service plans nationwide. In fact, Kimball's underling, Bryce Twitty, took a lead role in spreading the model. He traveled widely, meeting with fellow hospital administrators, employers, and union and civic leaders.[51] Yet having overcome the financial challenges, hospital service plans still faced formidable social and political hurdles before it could emerge as a national movement.

Having observed Baylor's success, two other Dallas-area hospitals quickly organized their own prepayment plans. Of course, this presented the specter of competition between hospitals and raised the ire of local physicians, who on occasion found that they lacked practice privileges at a hospital where their patients had prepaid benefits. The problem of competition proved far easier to solve than the growing resistance of doctors. In numerous metropolitan areas, multihospital service plans emerged that permitted beneficiaries to seek treatment at any member institution. In Sacramento, Durham, Washington, D.C., Cleveland, and Saint Paul, hospitals came together to jointly launch group prepayment plans along the lines of the original Baylor model. Surprisingly, the nationally recognized American Hospital Association (AHA) remained hesitant about the growing movement. In fact, it was a local organizer in Saint Paul, E. A. van Steenwyk, who created the symbol of a bold blue Geneva cross to publicize his area's plans. Soon thereafter, hospital service plans across the country adopted van Steenwyk's blue cross to represent their own plans, well before any formal Blue Cross organization existed. The AHA and the

American College of Physicians belatedly approved group hospitalization plans in 1934.

To regain the initiative, the AHA hired a former CCMC researcher, C. Rufus Rorem, to head up the AHA's Committee on Hospital Service. In 1938, with thirty-eight plans in existence and membership approaching 1.5 million, Rorem harnessed the Blue Cross plans into an associative relationship with the AHA. In exchange for its members accepting common standards, the AHA permitted its own logo to be used at the center of their blue cross, and more important, promised the political might of the AHA to defend them. Rorem described himself as a "safe man" in health care, a necessity if he was to succeed in managing the growth of Blue Cross.[52] Because hospital plans were nonprofit civil society organizations, critics occasionally tagged their leaders Communist, an irony given that the movement was inspired early on by industrialists and granted employers a powerful position. To a large extent, the name-calling resulted from doctors' anxiety about the future of U.S. medical care. Having defeated New Deal initiatives on government-directed health insurance, doctors now struggled to guard their professional sovereignty in the face of enterprising nonstate actors, including Blue Cross and group practices.

Blue Cross faced a thorny issue from its beginning: How to pay physicians whose care patients regarded as part of hospital services, namely, radiologists, pathologists, and anesthesiologists? Prior to prepayment plans, their bills had simply appeared with the other itemized hospital treatment charges. Now these physicians were asked to accept payment from a third party who, they felt, would inevitably seek to influence their practice of medicine. The various Blue Cross plans dealt with these in-hospital physicians in various ways, usually by billing patients separately or convincing the doctors to accept payment from the plan. Yet their basic complaint soon echoed throughout the medical profession. As Blue Cross expanded, patients and employers demanded an analogous institution to cover doctors' medical fees.

Medical leaders also faced rebellions against private fee-for-service medicine from within their own ranks. Innovative doctors struck out to create group practices that accepted prepayment of capitated medical fees, often in collaboration with local employers. In one of many such initiatives, Donald Ross and H. Clifford Loos entered into an agreement to provide comprehensive medical services to employees of the Los Angeles Department of Water and Power. By 1935, their clinic provided care to twelve thousand workers and twenty-five thousand dependents; membership cost $2.69 per month, less than half the average of what a comparable nonmember worker spent on health care. At about the same time, another doctor, Sidney Garfield, opened a group practice that served five thousand workers who were building an aqueduct across the California desert. Garfield would later join Henry J. Kaiser to build a massive system to deliver prepaid medical services at Kaiser's industrial complexes, and eventually, to the general public. Yet another threat to fee-for-service practice came from Oklahoma, where rural populism had inspired a local doctor, Michael Shadid, to create a medical cooperative that employed twenty general practitioners and specialists.

In each of these cases, the AMA responded with vitriolic attacks and backed local medical societies in their efforts to seek restrictive state legislation. These battles dragged on for years in state legislatures and in the courts. In the case of Shadid's cooperative, the AMA became exasperated when it learned that the powerful Oklahoma Farmers' Union was behind Shadid and that it had easily blocked their offensive against him in both the state legislature and the governor's office.[53] Whether these battles were won or lost, the lesson for AMA leaders was clear: to protect private-practice medicine, the profession itself must control voluntary insurance for medical services. In 1938, the AMA officially endorsed Blue Cross plans as long as "such plans do not incorporate medical services." What is more, medical leaders encouraged "local medical societies to develop plans in accordance with local needs" and, for the first time ever, endorsed voluntary "cash indemnity insurance for the payment of professional bills incurred during a prolonged or emergency illness providing such plans have the approval of the medical society concerned."[54] California served as the crucible in which this new policy directive took concrete form.

There a newly elected governor, Culbert Olson, had campaigned on the promise of compulsory health insurance financed by payroll deductions. In response, the California Medical Society organized the first medical society insurance plan, appropriating Blue Cross's now widely recognized royal blue color to create a shield emblazoned with a medical insignia. They called themselves "Blue Shield of California." Like Blue Cross, and in accordance with AMA principles, Blue Shield plans organized themselves as not-for-profit membership corporations, not insurance companies, and thereby escaped state insurance laws. This decision led to legal wrangling with Earl Warren, California's attorney general at the time, a conflict that would ultimately be settled in Blue Shield's favor by the U.S. Supreme Court.

For all their growing pains, and despite the occasionally testy relations between them, Blue Shield and Blue Cross ultimately succeeded because the New Deal had failed to offer any alternative. Employers and workers signed up in droves. In February 1940, fifty-two thousand Ford employees enrolled simultaneously in Blue Cross and Blue Shield. GM and Chrysler followed soon thereafter. By 1942, Blue Shield plans had 450,000 enrollees. As for doctors, even the most vociferous defenders of private-practice medicine soon accommodated themselves to a cash-rich third payer. John Mannix, an early Michigan Blue Shield administrator, described how the plan's staff made their Friday afternoon rounds in Flint with "very, very large sums of money [going] into doctors' offices and paying them in cash." John Castelucci, also a Michigan plan administrator and later a longtime president of the National Association of Blue Shield Plans, remarked, "It was an intrusion on their practice. But it was not an intrusion to take the money." During the Second World War, Blue Cross plans expanded at about 2 million enrollees per year to reach a total subscription of 24.2 million by 1947. Blue Shield plans started seven years later and experienced a much slower, albeit steady growth, reaching 4.4 million members by 1946.[55] In achieving greater coverage while defending private medicine and expanding physician sovereignty, the plans exhibited revealing similarities and contrasts with developments in France.

The Plight of Health Care Civil Society Organizations

A comparison of developments in the United States and France underlines just how influential private-practice medicine remained in both countries and the intrinsic differences between Blue Cross and Blue Shield. Most important, however, is that, in the absence of any explicit public policy or legislation, the most popular health care civil society organizations that Americans ever created, Blue Cross and Blue Shield, could not long survive as nonprofit service organizations. The meteoric rise of Blue Cross was due, in large part, to the intermediary role it played between citizens, their employers, and the market. Like the popularity of French mutual societies, this set the hospital service plans apart from private entrepreneurial initiatives and contributed greatly to their growth. A Cleveland Blue Cross official captured the public's enthusiasm for nonprofit hospital service plans in 1935, noting that "governors and mayors proclaimed Blue Cross enrollment periods, service clubs took part in promotion, Boy Scouts delivered enrollment material to prospects, and clergymen from the pulpit urged people to enroll in this community enterprise."[56]

Blue Cross plans shunned boards elected from among union members and rarely granted more than a token number of seats to union delegates.[57] Nevertheless, as noninvestor-owned organizations, these plans included a sufficiently diverse group of leaders to build public confidence in their commitment to community service. According to the 1937 agreement that created the national Blue Cross Association, plans agreed to divide seats on their governing boards among hospital officials, medical professionals, and members of the general public. They further agreed to continue their nonprofit standing, flatly stating that "no private investors should provide money as stockholders or owners."[58] These pledges, alongside the striking growth of numerous plans in working-class communities, lent a grassroots character to Blue Cross that permitted its leaders to shrug off criticism that sought to label the movement Communist.

Put differently, much like French mutual societies, Blue Cross plans could get away with socializing the cost of hospital care in a society otherwise fearful of collectivist initiatives in medical care because of their status as civil society organizations. In both the United States and France, physicians were suspicious of the movements' expansion into medical services, fearing for their professional sovereignty, which they viewed as inextricably bound up with individual practitioners' direct collection of fees. Herein we see the extent to which Blue Cross made the creation of Blue Shield inevitable.

U.S. physicians, having effectively fought any New Deal promulgation of compulsory health insurance, could not long look the other way as the public demanded a socialization of the costs of medical services to complement hospital service plans. In this light, the growth of Shadid's Oklahoma health co-op and the Ross-Loos group practices in Los Angeles were clear symptoms of unmet public demands, which medical leaders ignored at their peril. These early experiments in the prepayment of medical services served as a wake-up call for the AMA, much as the restrictive German-style health insurance methods of Alsace-Lorraine had for French medical leaders a decade earlier. U.S. and French medical leaders, both of whom were deeply committed to private-practice medicine, realized that the surest way to protect it would be to draw up the rules under which insurers lived.

Because of their nonprofit status, the Blue Shield plans, sanctioned by medical societies, enjoyed much the same public enthusiasm as that which propelled Blue Cross memberships. Even though Blue Shield plans could not claim anywhere near the same populist origins as the hospital plans, workers, employers, and the general public granted them similar trust.

Quite simply, physicians began selling group health insurance policies to evade the intrusion of laypeople into the administration of medical services. Indeed, it might appear that U.S. physicians had bested their French colleagues in the battle to defend private-practice fee-for-service medicine. Instead of turning to the state to protect their professional sovereignty, as French physicians had done by agreeing to a compromise on compulsory health insurance in 1930, U.S. physicians, through their medical society–anointed Blue Shield plans, had *become* the country's most important health insurers. Yet without the statutory protections that French doctors enjoyed, and without a political consensus on the proper role of insurers that guided French mutual societies, Blue Shield and Blue Cross soon found themselves under attack from the commercial insurance industry.

The inspiration for this attack lay in the very inventiveness of the Blues' success and the absence of any government health policy to prevent it. Blue Cross and then Blue Shield abandoned traditional practices whereby insurers calculated different prices for different groups, what is known as *experience rating*, based on the age, sex, occupation, and other relevant criteria of the purchasing groups. Instead, the Blues sold all their group policies at one *community rate*, ignoring information on which commercial insurers had long depended to price their products. In and of itself, community rating was not untenable. The Blues confidently relied on the pooling of high- and low-risk beneficiaries to create a single, heterogeneous mix of subscribers, to whom they could offer an affordable price. Under community rating, healthy workers inevitably subsidized the medical expenses of their sicker and less lucky fellows—an outcome that many viewed as inherently equitable. The Blues' community rating mirrored the approach of compulsory health insurance in France. All participants fell into the same pool for comprehensive hospital and medical services. As long as an insurer is alone in the market, community rating has an enviable actuarial soundness and administrative simplicity.

By the late 1940s, commercial insurers had studied the success and actuarial data of group health insurance sufficiently to allow them to effectively enter into competition with the Blues. They brought their well-honed skills of risk assessment, which they used to offer lower premiums to firms that employed workers who were healthier than average and presented less risk. Employers, after all, were in business to make money, and found the lower premiums irresistible. As some of them switched to commercial insurers' experience-rated policies, they left behind costlier-than-average workers in Blue Cross and Blue Shield insurance pools. To compensate, the Blues raised premiums, but this only encouraged more finely-tuned experience rating from the commercials who, because of the Blues' premium hikes, found additional groups to which they could offer relatively lower prices. A vicious cycle set in whereby community rating, without the statutory protections that existed in France, became financially untenable.

By the late 1950s, the Blues had little choice but to abandon community rating in favor of experience-rated policies, a first step for many plans in an inexorable march toward converting to for-profit corporations and becoming largely indistinguishable from commercial insurers. To be sure, the Blues long maintained their commitment to public service, but commercial insurers increasingly viewed their missionary zeal as sanctimonious and ultimately irrelevant. In the absence of New Deal action on health insurance and the erosion of Blue Cross and Blue Shield as civil society intermediaries, hospital and medical services came increasingly to be viewed no differently from other insurable risks such as fire or theft.

Despite their pioneering efforts, leaders of the Blues proved ideologically incapable of imagining measures by which they might preserve their plans as nonprofit civil society organizations. One exception may have been none other than Blue Cross's champion at the American Hospital Association, C. Rufus Rorem. Rorem clashed early with Cleveland Hospital Association leader John McNamara, especially after Rorem proclaimed that the principal purpose of Blue Cross plans should be to "solve the problems of the individual and *the public* who own the hospitals," a comment that apparently sounded too Marxist for some in the Blue Cross leadership. It seems that Rorem never shook the reputation he acquired from having worked for the CCMC, whose majority report in 1932 had advocated consideration of compulsory health insurance. Growing suspicions that Rorem viewed Blue Cross as a successful experiment in health security but also believed that government intervention would ultimately be necessary to sustain its growth led McNamara to accuse Rorem of being a Communist and to call an emergency meeting of Blue Cross directors to consider the charges. Rorem survived the inquisition but resigned shortly thereafter at the age of fifty, seemingly at the height of his career. Other Blue Cross leaders persevered in their attachment to voluntary insurance. As one put it, Blue Cross saw itself as a part of "the long struggle to keep hospital insurance a voluntary venture."[59]

Although a commitment to equality lay behind the Blues' policy of community-rated premiums, their "dogmatic privatism" and individualistic notions of liberty ultimately determined their fate in the rapidly changing

4

CHALLENGES AND CHANGE DURING THE SECOND WORLD WAR, 1940–1945

Call it socialized medicine or what you will, it is helping a lot of farm families to get the best medical care they ever had, and that in the face of a wartime shortage of doctors.

> Arkansas physician, commenting on the Farm Security Administration's health care program during the Second World War

In May 1940 German forces launched their long-planned blitzkrieg against France. The French army, backed by a British expeditionary force, was quickly split in two by the fast-moving German tank divisions and aerial attacks. With supply and communications lines disrupted, the Nazi advance quickly turned into a rout. Only an unusually dense fog over the English Channel prevented the total destruction of the fleeing French army and their British allies. Six weeks later, the troops of what many had regarded as the most formidable army in Europe sat helplessly in German prisoner-of-war camps or had already fled to Britain. As the Germans advanced, France's republican government retreated to the southwestern port city of Bordeaux. There, in a fateful vote on 10 July 1940, Parliament elevated the country's most respected general of the First World War, Philippe Pétain, to head of state, effectively dissolving France's democracy. Pétain immediately sought an armistice with Germany and established a new government in the central spa town of Vichy.

The calamitous defeat of June invoked a deep introspection among the French, who were bewildered by their sudden fall from national greatness. Pétain insisted that the cause of France's defeat lay in the selfish individualism and degenerate social values of the republic. Pétain therefore called for a "National Revolution" to restore the honor and dignity of the nation, a reformation that included important changes to health care.

Doctors first felt the heavy hand of Pétain's Vichy regime in July 1940, when the government took control of their medical association headquarters and handed it over to a newly created physicians' group, the Ordre des Médecins (Order of doctors). In fact, the Vichy state abolished all professional organizations and independent workers' unions. In their place, the government created "organizational committees" in preparation for what historians call "corporatism." Under corporatism, diverse groups such as workers and employers cooperate under government supervision for the common good. The new employers' association, like its republican predecessor, wielded significant influence, but workers and professionals had to settle for organizations bereft of the power to strike. The new Ordre des Médecins dictated that physicians reconceive their associational life and move away from the customary practice whereby their *syndicats* expressed physicians' collective interest vis-à-vis the state and society. In exchange, the order promised to enforce doctors' sovereignty over medical ethics, education, research, licensure, and public health.[1]

Yet the order demonstrated different priorities than the CSMF it replaced. Its first governing board boded ill for private fee-for-service medicine, tilting instead toward state-directed approaches to medical care. Of twelve members, only three were private practitioners; the other nine hailed from public hospitals or university medical schools. Under the republic, by contrast, the medical leadership had reflected the demographic of most of the country's doctors, who were in private practice. These generalists and specialists were by far the most ardent defenders of fee-for-service practice. The first president of the Ordre des Médecins, René Leriche, summed up Vichy's critique of the republic and the old medical association, when he warned that "our desire for independence ... must not result in an individualism that would stoke anarchy and disorder, making it impossible for us to comprehend today's demands."[2] Leriche urged doctors to cultivate conformity and respect at a time of national crisis.

Almost immediately after its creation, the Ordre des Médecins set about redrafting the physicians' Code of Ethics under the guidance of Vichy's minister of public health and family, Serge Huard. The new code included forceful language in defense of private-practice medicine.[3] But when the doctors sought to use it against recalcitrant mutual society clinics, they obtained little cooperation from Vichy officials. More troublesome still, doctors themselves split over the future of their profession. Prestigious physicians came forward to support Vichy's social medicine initiatives. Some even called private medical practice and fee-for-service medicine obsolete. Marc Nédélec urged his colleagues to adopt "a new medicine... that accounts for the social, economic, and technological era in which we live... From this point of view, the medical Charter [which contained legal protections for private-practice medicine] is outmoded and must be revised." Nédélec called for the abandonment of patients' direct payment of fees, limitations on a patient's choice of physician, and modifications in the medical confidentiality law. The result, he argued, would be far more modern and egalitarian health care that benefited doctors and patients alike.[4] Although Nédélec's call was heretical to old guard medical leaders, enough physicians equivocated that Vichy officials could claim doctors were divided on the importance of private medical practice.

Vichy employed doctors to inspect schools and workplaces, a duty usually reserved for private practitioners. The regime also enacted reforms that opened more hospitals to the general public, a change that had long been stalled under the republic because it threatened private practitioners' business. Reform of hospitals reinforced their public character, sanctioned a new national medical fee structure for treatment, and fully integrated doctors onto hospital staffs. Without a doubt, these reforms accelerated the transformation of hospitals from hostels for the destitute and chronically ill into centers of advanced medical care for the general population. But by far Vichy's most enduring health care initiatives focused on improving the country's population growth rate, especially in rural France.

Pétain repeatedly blamed France's calamitous defeat on the demographic frailty caused by decadence and degeneracy in the nation's cities. Concerns about low population growth and an emphasis on the importance of hardy farm families to the nation's vitality were hardly new in 1940. Since the late nineteenth century, political leaders and publicists had often extolled family farmers as the keel of the nation. This veneration gained further credence during the First World War, when rural villages supplied most of the infantry regiments that fought on the western front. The tragic loss of these men—often fathers along with their sons—are memorialized in thousands of town squares throughout the country. To atone for and replace these losses, natalists fueled the public's reverence for farm families throughout the 1920s and 1930s, obtaining greatly expanded benefits for rural families under social insurance and family welfare laws. Vichy bolstered these and launched new initiatives of its own to improve rural health standards and to encourage women to have more children.

The regime exalted motherhood as a woman's national duty. Mothers of twelve or more children received national medals and personal letters from Pétain, who celebrated their children as proof that France would survive. The government tightly restricted the dissemination of information about effective birth control methods and devices. Abortion was outlawed and abortionists subjected to capital punishment, a law that resulted in the execution of one woman in 1943. Alongside curbs on reproductive information and rights, women faced limitations on gainful employment, which Vichy officials considered a distraction from motherhood and domesticity.[5] Vichy's prescription for women represented the apotheosis of maternalist health policy founded on a notion of *republican motherhood*, a philosophy that was also widely embraced in the nineteenth-century United States. It granted women a privileged status as bearers of male citizens but denied women suffrage and other fundamental civil rights that would have translated into full-fledged citizenship.[6]

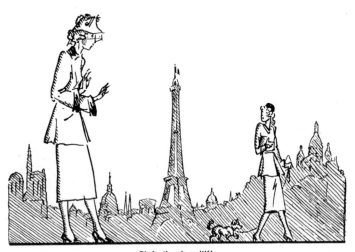

Diminution de moitié!
1.000 Parisiennes ne mettent au monde que 500 filles pour les remplacer à la génération suivante.

Figure 2. Illustration in a typical natalist tract from the late 1930s attacking the barrenness of cities relative to the countryside. The caption reads: "Half as Much! One thousand Parisian women produce only five hundred girls to replace the next generation." Fernand Boverat, "Comment nous vaincrons la dénatalité" (Paris: Editions de l'Alliance Nationale Contre la Dépopulation, 1939), 10.

Having stripped women of their economic and reproductive rights, France's wartime government sought to assure the success of women's pregnancies for the sake of the nation's population growth. Thus was born the country's impressive network of free prenatal, well-baby, and pediatric clinics, collectively known as PMI Centers (Centres de Protection Maternelle Infantile). In time, these centers would drive down infant mortality rates to levels seen in few other places in the world. The regime simultaneously introduced a *carnet de santé*, a compulsory record of all vaccinations, immunizations, growth milestones, and illnesses, which parents were required to have and maintain. The *carnet de santé* represented only a minor intrusion on the physician's usual record keeping. The PMI centers, however, represented a significant expansion of the state's role in health care. Women could not choose their doctors and state authorities paid practitioners directly, not the patient. Private practitioners' loss of clout during the war did not go unnoticed by France's mutual movement.

Their national leaders engaged the Vichy regime as a partner from the beginning. They sought a renewal of the fight they had lost over the expansion of mutual society–run medical facilities in the early 1930s. Mutual federation leader Romain Laveille suggested that "the principal difficulties which have arisen between the mutual movement and doctors are their code of ethics . . . which opposes any hindrance to the free choice [of doctor] . . . and refuses any regulations that would force adherence to a third-payer system." Another mutual leader added that physicians "have succeeded in creating a privileged situation based on their important services and on purely material interests." At their 1943 meeting, the national mutual federation approved a series of hard-hitting resolutions, including one that charged doctors with "abusive practices" and labeled "unacceptable a doctor's judgment of a patient's condition in the sole pursuit of augmenting his personal profit." Other resolutions dubbed doctors' rate increases unfair and called for the spread of contract medical practices.[7]

Just when it appeared that private-practice medicine would not survive the onslaught of Vichy directives and mutual society designs, large-scale fighting returned to France, with salutary effects for a renewal of fee-for-service private-practice medicine. In July 1944, as Allied troops pushed out from the beaches of Normandy, aided by coordinated French Resistance attacks, German commanders ordered that all French doctors immediately report to German authorities any treatment provided to wounded Resistance fighters. At great personal risk, the president of the Ordre des Médecins, Louis Portes, countermanded the German order. In an emergency mailing to all physicians, Portes reminded his colleagues that they "have no other responsibility than to treat the wounded, respect for medical confidentiality being essential to the patient's confidence in his doctor. There exists no administrative objective that should violate it."[8] This defiant act marked the first step in rebuilding an independent French medical profession and revived doctors' solidarity in protecting private medicine after the war.

The Vichy government was driven from power by Allied armies in August 1944. During its tenure, it had failed to correct one of the single greatest quandaries in French health security: the continued inadequacy of reimbursement of medical bills for workers subject to the country's health insurance law. In fact, with the notable exception of Vichy's hospital reform law, the Free French planners, hard at work in London preparing for the reestablishment of the republic, regarded most of Vichy's social policy "so imbued with reactionary thinking that it is difficult to lend the slightest confidence to the entire edifice that has been so painstakingly created by the 'hinterland' authorities at Vichy." Corporatism, which banned workers' unions, came in for especially harsh criticism; it was called an "indescribable muddle of medieval rules that challenges all good sense and logic . . . [its] entire construction is based uniquely on force and therefore doomed in advance."[9] Free French planners sympathized with Vichy's efforts to aid rural families and to shore up the country's birth rate, but the return of the republic would bring female suffrage and a sharp rejection of Vichy's extreme conservatism on women's role in society.

U.S. Government Health Care Programs during the Second World War

With France under German occupation and an authoritarian government, one might suppose that French health care policy diverged more widely than ever from its U.S. counterpart. The French republic had been overthrown and civil rights suspended. Meanwhile, Americans successfully defended their democracy, separated, as Thomas Jefferson once noted, "by nature and a wide ocean from the exterminating havoc of one quarter of the globe."[10] Indeed, the United States stood as a great moral force for the nation's soldiers now fighting in Europe and in the Pacific. Still millions more, who suffered under the yoke of German and Japanese oppression, looked to the United States for hope and liberation. Yet the vast moral divide between Vichy and Washington should not blind us to several striking parallels in the realm of health care. These parallels lay in government health programs and were made possible by the state's greatly expanded role in both countries. What is more, the inspirations for state action emanated from shared ideals concerning the nation's source and sustenance, namely, children and the countryside.

Just as Vichy created its mother and children's health clinics, the United States pursued an extraordinary expansion of maternal and well-baby clinics during the war. Assistant Chief of the Children's Bureau Martha Eliot won a wholesale expansion of the Emergency Maternity and Infant Care program (EMIC) in 1940. She seized on the displacement caused by military mobilization, which affected thousands of married couples in their prime child-bearing years. Because of forced relocation, women were without familiar health care practitioners or the family members who normally supported them during pregnancy and after the births of their children. The nation's future citizens, argued Eliot, were clearly at risk.

Under EMIC, servicemen's wives received prenatal, delivery, and post-partum care from a hospital of their choice, as well as well-baby services until the child reached one year of age. Although the program was restricted to the four lowest military pay grades, wartime conscription and recruitment had so expanded the armed forces that the wives of 75 percent of the navy and of 87 percent of army personnel were eligible. By 1944, the Children's Bureau announced, EMIC paid for one out of seven births nationally and operated in all but four states and Puerto Rico.[11] For many of these women, EMIC permitted their first-ever access to hospital treatment and, like Blue Cross, represented a major departure in the mode of payment for hospital and accompanying medical services. AMA leaders conceded that EMIC placed the profession in "an intolerable dilemma." Opposition to improved medical care access for military families would have appeared "unpatriotic"—a byword that AMA propagandists knew all too well because they themselves had repeatedly used it in their campaigns against compulsory health insurance. Finding prudence the better side of valor, the AMA held its fire against EMIC until the circumstances had changed.[12] But EMIC constituted only one of the two wartime government-directed health care programs.

As in France, the other served the countryside. Here too, proponents rightfully pointed to the Depression and wartime exigencies to justify the expansion of Farm Security Administration (FSA) health care services. Although the FSA was far from the only New Deal relief agency involved in medical care, it was the largest, and by a great deal. By 1942 the FSA had created twelve hundred medical plans in forty-one states, had enrolled

650,000 poor rural inhabitants, and operated in more than a third of all counties in the country.[13] Its procedures varied from region to region, but in general, the FSA adopted a community-centered approach that respected local private practitioners, creating voluntary health insurance cooperatives in the hardest-hit regions. Ably led by some of the most committed New Deal reformers, the FSA succeeded at a time when New Deal health insurance initiatives were under daily attack from Congress and the public. As the FSA historian Michael Grey notes, "In his second inaugural address in 1937, President Roosevelt spoke of one third of a nation as 'ill-housed, ill-clad, and ill-nourished.' The FSA learned that . . . many poor rural families were just plain ill."[14]

Early on, the FSA was invulnerable to political assault because of the sheer need in the rural areas. Drought and depression brought destitution to vast swathes of the Great Plains states, the Southwest, California, and the South. In 1932 alone, 60 percent of the farms in North Dakota were sold to pay creditors and a third of the state's population depended on county welfare to survive. The utter poverty of farm communities made them actuarially unattractive to health insurers, even nonprofit service plans such as Blue Cross, let alone commercial companies. In 1941, when fully 20 percent of urban families enjoyed some sort of health coverage, only 3 percent of rural families could say the same. As late as 1947, when Blue Cross enrolled its 24 millionth member, only 1.6 percent of its subscribers hailed from the countryside. In the same year, the proportion was somewhat better among Blue Shield plans, but still only 7 percent of total enrollees.[15]

Demand for FSA-subsidized health cooperatives emerged not only from the unmet medical needs of poor farmers but also from the grim circumstances of rural practitioners. In the dust bowl states, physicians' incomes fell 50 percent during the Depression. Nationally, rural doctors' collections fell from 75 percent of billed services in the 1920s to about 40 percent after 1929.[16] After the outbreak of the war, military recruitment reduced the countryside's already meager medical contingent. Thus, when FSA officials arrived in one rural county after another after 1935 and offered to pay struggling physicians to care for their needy neighbors, they found many willing participants. Equally important, the FSA paid between 60 and 90 percent of customary fees, depending on the procedure, and respected doctors' private medical practices, including a patient's choice of physician.

Medical leaders at AMA headquarters in Chicago turned a deaf ear to the cries of help from their rural colleagues. The AMA Judicial Council insisted that all doctors uphold "the age-old professional ideal of medical service to all, whether able to pay or not." The council further charged that those who collaborated with the FSA were taking "the greatest step toward socialized medicine…which the medical profession could take."[17] Rural practitioners' response to this admonition was not at all what AMA leaders expected.

Country doctors across the nation filled the pages of their local medical journals with stinging indictments of the AMA.[18] As one Arkansas physician put it, "I'm for the program 100 percent. Call it socialized medicine or what you will, it is helping a lot of farm families to get the best medical care they ever had, and that in the face of a wartime shortage of doctors."[19] To be sure, rural doctors had a material interest in the FSA, which partly explains their support. But material interest alone cannot fully explain the rage that rural practitioners heaped on their national leaders. Nor can it explain the FSA's ability to fight off calls for its elimination in Congress after the midterm elections of 1938, when conservative Democrats joined Republicans in attacks against the FSA and many other New Deal social programs.

As in the case of the French wartime government's focus on rural communities, to fully explain the success of the FSA, one must consider the cultural ideal of rural America. Family farmers who were devastated by the Depression and then freely gave up their sons for military service during the war embodied the most "authentic" Americans for residents of city and countryside alike. They served as living reminders of the frontier pioneers who had wrestled with nature, pushing the boundaries of the original colonies and then the fledgling republic farther and farther west. Ironically, the ancestors of these "authentic Americans" (with the help of the U.S. Army) had dispossessed indigenous peoples of their land in order to attain their idealized status. Indeed, gender and race played an important role in the FSA's image. Although the agency aided many African American and Latino families, Dorothea Lange's photo of a mother with three young children, *Migrant Mother*, and Walker Evans's montage of white Alabama sharecroppers became the most widely circulated representations of FSA beneficiaries, perhaps even of all New Deal social relief recipients. The subjects of these photos and their appeal back in Washington were no coincidence. It was not until the late 1970s the public learned that the subject of Lange's photograph was, in fact, Cherokee.[20]

In a phrase that is still salient today, farmers represented "the heartland," which was not just a geographical place but a psychological and cultural ideal that remained essentially white. Moreover, farmers were, according to the ideal, untouched by the decadence of burgeoning metropolises. In a

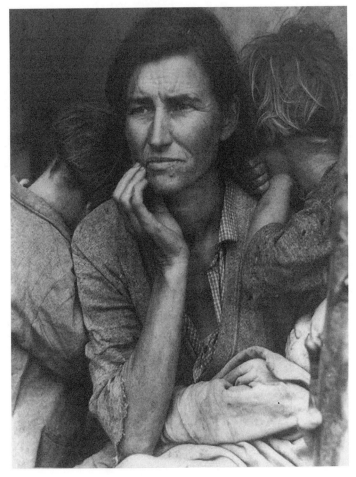

Figure 3. Migrant Mother. Photograph by Dorothea Lange, Farm Security Administration, 1936. Library of Congress, Farm Security Administration, LC-USF34-009058-C [P&P].

larger sense, rural America represented a haven—a refuge in both physical and psychological terms—removed from the total war in which the nation was then engaged. When AMA leaders in Chicago accused their poor rural colleagues of caving in to Socialism, that is, to a foreign ideal, rural doctors in essence shot back that nothing could be more authentic and important than the health of the American farm family. After all, the beneficiaries of FSA health care cooperatives produced the nation's food supply during a time of national emergency, a fact that FSA advocates used with great effect to answer their critics in Congress. Like France's infant and child welfare clinics, the

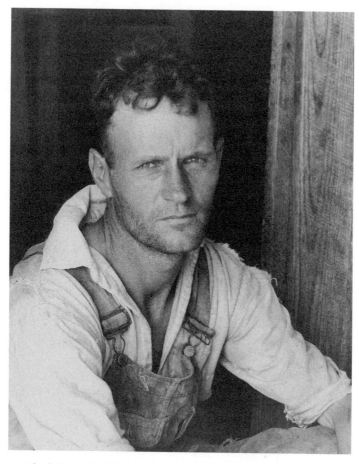

Figure 4. Floyd Burroughs, Sharecropper. Photograph by Walker Evans, Farm Security Administration, 1936. Library of Congress, Farm Security Administration, LC-USF342-T01-008138-A.

FSA enjoyed a shield of cultural veneration that both inspired and protected its actions.

What ultimately undermined the FSA and EMIC was U.S. economic recovery, which was accompanied by renewed efforts to enact government-sponsored health insurance. By early 1941, unemployment was dropping by one percentage point a month. Nationally, wages rose on average 20 percent in the following year. As the improving economic conditions slowly spread to the countryside, physicians there reacted much the same way as French doctors when the end of the war was in sight. As their practices improved, they rediscovered their faith in private-practice medicine, and as a result, the dangers of the FSA to their professional sovereignty.

In 1943 Senator Robert Wagner of New York, Senator James Murray of Montana, and representative John Dingell of Michigan launched another effort to enact compulsory health insurance. Once again, Franklin Roosevelt demurred, refusing to invest presidential prestige in the campaign. The Wagner-Murray-Dingell proposal, which was quickly dubbed WMD, represented the country's first truly national health insurance legislation, since the federal government played a dominant role. Unlike Wagner's 1939 attempt, WMD foresaw little role for the states. Instead, the bill opened a new chapter in the Social Security Act of 1935, offering medical and hospitalization coverage to all old age insurance beneficiaries and their dependents.

In language reminiscent of the AALL bill of 1916, WMD set up open panels of physicians from whom patients could choose their general practitioners. It also left the method of payment for medical services for the local doctors to decide. They could continue with fee-for-service private medicine, create capitated schemes, accept full- or part-time salaries, or combine these methods in various ways. WMD granted administrative powers over the entire system to the U.S. surgeon general, including the certification of local physician panels and negotiations with participating hospitals. To pay for the new health care benefits, WMD levied a 12 percent payroll tax, divided equally between employer and employee, on the first three thousand dollars of earned income.[21]

With the introduction of WMD, Farm Security Administration leaders realized that their fourteen thousand field agents occupied a pivotal position between local medical societies and the federal government, one that could be crucial in rallying rural support for the bill. They took heart in their knowledge that many rural physicians understood that large portions of their practices were not actuarially sound enough to ever attract purely voluntary forms of health insurance to the countryside. Thus the FSA openly backed national health insurance, producing educational pamphlets and seeking to garner the support of rural medical societies.

The AMA's reaction was swift and effective. Its leaders took delight in accusing "the FSA of disguising its real agenda all along."[22] Once FSA leaders had openly entered the political fray, their legitimacy as relief agents devoted to the country's heartland came under attack. One after another, state medical societies where the FSA had cultivated strong working partnerships called on their county affiliates to refuse further cooperation.

Meanwhile, although WMD attracted the support of the nation's largest unions, including the Congress of Industrial Organizations (CIO) and the American Federation of Labor (AFL), it died in committee in 1943.[23] As for the FSA, after several debilitating cuts, it was finally eliminated in 1946.

Toward the end of the war, the Emergency Maternal and Infant Care program (EMIC) also attached itself to new federal health care legislation, with a similar result: it drew deadly counterfire from physicians, health insurers, and even the administration's own Social Security Bureau. EMIC's initial appeal stemmed from its conservative goal of aiding displaced servicemen's wives in their maternal role. Yet when EMIC leader Martha Eliot joined with Senator Claude Pepper of Florida to draft a postwar program for women and children's health care, the resulting bill was a major departure from both the employer-based approach advocated by the Social Security Bureau and traditional child-centered poverty relief. Pepper's Maternal and Child Welfare bill stipulated that health care was a right for pregnant women and children. Women need not have paid payroll taxes or be a dependent of someone who did (as under WMD) to be eligible. Nor would they be subjected to any sort of means test.

The Pepper bill, despite being restricted to mothers and their young children, was philosophically much closer to a British-style national health service than anything else ever proposed in the United States. Funding came from general tax revenues, and physicians were to be paid on a capitated or salaried basis for participation in group practices, clinics, and hospitals. Fee-for-service practice would be used only as a last resort.[24] Like FSA leaders in rural America, Pepper and EMIC leaders sought to capitalize on a cultural ideal that privileged women and children as the most deserving recipients of a specialized health care system. EMIC leader Elliot hoped that the Pepper bill would serve as a wedge for establishing universal health coverage that dispensed with both the strictures of fee-for-service medicine and reliance on workplace payrolls. Such a bold initiative, however, drew opposition not only from the AMA and health insurers; it also found scant support from within the Roosevelt administration or among labor leaders because it departed so radically from the model of employment-based health security that had taken hold in the 1930s and became entrenched during the war.[25]

The Wartime Boost to Employment-Based Health Security

Government programs for maternal, child, and rural health stood side by side with U.S. labor's pursuit of health insurance at the collective bargaining table. In contrast to the situation in Vichy France, corporatism succeeded in the United States. U.S. labor leaders made a no-strike pledge in January 1942, obtaining in return Roosevelt's promise to create a National War Labor Board (NWLB) to assure their equitable treatment by employers. Labor's no-strike pledge was not entirely uncoerced, however. Congress was then deliberating on how to make strikes in war industries illegal and was even considering a bill that would have forced industrial workers into government service. The origins of the NWLB notwithstanding, its arbitration of disputes over worker compensation in the war industries shaped labor and management attitudes on health care and third-party payers in ways that would endure for decades to come.

The National War Labor Board's principal goal was to assure production, that is, to avoid strikes, and to hold inflation to an absolute minimum—no mean feat in a wartime economy operating at full capacity. Under normal conditions, employers and workers often avoid strikes through wage increases, but wartime corporatism foreclosed strikes, and wage hikes were tightly circumscribed to avoid inflation. This left so-called fringe benefits as much-needed lubricant for collective bargaining during the war. Unions successfully obtained concessions from employers on health insurance because the NWLB believed that nonwage compensation was less likely to cause inflation. As the historian Jennifer Klein notes, however, any liberties that the NWLB might have granted on health insurance were, when all was said and done, much less important than the message to labor unions that health security objectives should be "included in a labor-management contract, as a concession [to be] extracted from management."[26]

Labor leaders insisted that voluntary health insurance was a stopgap measure until they could win the legislative battle for national health insurance. They reasoned that if employers had already agreed to pay for health insurance at the collective bargaining table, they would be less likely to fight a law making it compulsory.[27] This may have been true, but it ignores the effect of private health insurance coverage on the rank and file. Workers could rightly ask: Why work for a federal law that would make us pay half the cost of health insurance when the boss now pays it all?

Moreover, when AFL and CIO leaders accepted voluntary insurance, they granted an extraordinary trust to third-party payers. Here we see the critical importance of Blue Cross and Blue Shield as civil society organizations. Union leaders lent more trust to the Blues than to commercial insurers because of their nonprofit status. Labor leaders were further lured by the tax-free aspect of health insurance benefits purchased under employers' group plans. When New Deal efforts to add health care to Social Security were convincingly blocked by the AMA and a conservative Congress, labor leaders readily embraced private health insurance as a solution.

Wartime corporatism provided the last required push. It put health security squarely on the collective bargaining table, and the NWLB sternly taught labor leaders and employers alike that health insurance belonged there. The embrace of private health insurance by both labor and management spurred a remarkable growth in coverage. By 1945, 32 million Americans were in a group health plan of some kind, more than half of them in Blue Cross. By 1950 fully 95 percent of CIO members had health care plans in their labor contracts.[28] Yet this progress only re-created a twentieth-century version of nineteenth-century health care inequality. Stably employed and especially unionized white men gained access to health security at far greater rates than (nondependent) women and minorities, especially those who worked in unorganized agricultural and service sectors.

Health care initiatives on behalf of rural inhabitants and women were inspired by ideals shared to a remarkable degree in France and the United States during the war, but the wartime takeoff of employment-based private health insurance in the United States marked a decisive divergence between the two nations. After 1945, health security in the United States became increasingly a privately provided good, with the government occasionally stepping in with supplemental initiatives. In France, an opposite dynamic developed. After the war, basic health security was increasingly viewed as a public good that should be guaranteed by the state. Private insurers were to provide supplemental coverage when and where government programs fell short. In both countries, private fee-for-service medicine survived the war intact, a testament to its tenacity in the face of unprecedented national upheavals.

5

LABOR'S QUEST FOR HEALTH SECURITY, 1945–1960

The Steelworkers believe that Blue Shield has lost sight of its original purpose and has deteriorated into a collection agency for the medical profession.

United Steelworkers Spokesman John Tomayko, 1957

Like two sides of the same coin, health care in France and the United States exhibited different images after 1945. The French side portrayed public compulsory health insurance with mutual societies and private insurers providing supplemental coverage for employers and individuals who could pay for it. The U.S. side showed the power of private voluntary insurance to afford comprehensive health security to millions, with compulsory public programs intervening only to cover some who were left out. Also like a single coin, the currency of health care in France and the United States remained the same. Political leaders, workers, employers, doctors, and insurers in both countries remained intrinsically attached to private-practice medicine and wage-funded health insurance premiums. These common traits, as much as the differences between the two nations on the issue of compulsion versus voluntarism, determined the evolution of health care in France and the United States after the Second World War.

We begin with France to explain why and how the nation turned to greatly expanded social insurance programs, especially *Sécurité Sociale*, created in 1945. Prepared by Resistance planners in London and implemented after the cessation of hostilities, *Sécurité Sociale* marked a milestone on the road to widespread health security, even though universal coverage would not be achieved until 2000. The personalities, politics, and psychology of its founding are therefore worth our sustained attention, especially because they differed so radically from developments in the United States.

War's end brought much change to U.S. social questions, yet developments in U.S. health care were relatively evolutionary. Political circumstances in the United States favored private voluntary health insurance. In fact, wartime developments in the United States undermined the chances of federal health care legislation. Opinion polls showed a sharp drop in support for national health insurance, due in large part to the spread of private, employment-based coverage. Further, AMA leaders painted those who advocated adding health insurance to Social Security as participants, naïve or knowing, in a Communist plot to overthrow U.S. democracy, a slanderous charge that even many physicians ultimately denounced, but not before it had helped turn public opinion against "socialized medicine." Even when there was no longer any chance for passage of national health insurance under President Harry Truman, AMA president Elmer Henderson smugly said its backers had a "pinkish pigmentation," thereby charging them with un-American activities.[1]

What a great contrast with France, where Communists were enjoying a surge in popularity because of their effectiveness as Resistance fighters against the German occupation. Communist leaders urged a revolutionary makeover of French society, including health care. Yet France's *Sécurité Sociale*, for all its noble goals and reordering of health care actors and interests, hardly constituted a revolutionary counterpoint to the U.S. case. It preserved far too many of the contradictions between the liberty of medical practice and equal access to health care.

Planning for *Sécurité Sociale*

Long before D-Day in June 1944, when hundreds of thousands of Allied soldiers invaded German-occupied France to begin their long march to Berlin, a distinguished group of French social reformers had been meeting regularly at 3 St. James Square, London. Henry Hauck, labor minister of the Free French under Charles de Gaulle, and Jean Gendrot led the assembly. Both men had been officials in the leftist workers' union, the Confédération Générale du Travail (CGT). Also working on postwar social planning was a high public official, Pierre Laroque. After his arrival in London in late 1942, Laroque quickly emerged as a powerful figure in de Gaulle's organization.[2] He had served in a key labor ministry position during the implementation of social insurance during the 1930s. In the wake of France's defeat, Laroque worked briefly for the Vichy labor ministry before being forced from government service because of his Jewish ancestry. Subsequently recruited by the Resistance, Laroque established a strong rapport with de Gaulle, whom he found receptive to a wholesale reform of health insurance.

Laroque, Gendrot, Hauck, and their colleagues examined the entirety of France's social protections as well as a broad array of political and economic issues they deemed likely to surface in postwar France. These included the government's role in economic planning, the nationalization of industries, worker participation in industrial management, and wage equity between men and women. Free French social planners clearly had an expansive view of social reform that included women in their own right and not merely as dependents of men.[3]

In contrast to the United States and most of the rest of Europe, France had failed to enact female suffrage between the world wars. Wartime planners clearly regarded the absence of women's civil equality as a hindrance to their plans for increased social protections. They condemned the "sociological conception of 'man, head of household,'" thereby opening the way for men and children to derive employment-based social insurance benefits from their employed wives or mothers.[4] The gender construction of man's role as head of household had led to widespread wage inequities and the denial of benefits to deserving families under the 1930 social insurance law.

French leaders continued their quest to increase the population growth rate after the war, and natalists remained influential in social policymaking.[5] But value-laden prescriptions for family policy, which implicitly blamed women for the country's low birthrate, reached their zenith under Vichy, never to return. In fact, women's suffrage was among the first decrees announced by de Gaulle's Provisional Government after the Liberation in 1944. Not only did wartime planners' attention to women symbolize a move toward gender equality, it also marked a renewed enthusiasm for interdependent citizenship writ large, since, alongside their discussion of women's civil rights and wage equity, London-based planners embraced universal health security.

The compulsory health insurance law of 1930 had never foreseen such an eventuality. Even its most ardent backers shied away from promoting it as a first step on the road to universal health care. *Solidaristes* before the war had wanted to avoid class conflict by giving the most vulnerable workers a modicum of health, wage, and retirement security. They had never advocated, for example, that public insurance funds pay the medical bills of well-to-do middle- and upper-income workers. Now planners in critical posts openly expressed their view that postliberation France should embody a vastly enlarged sense of solidarity that included all citizens of the restored republic. The new ethos, which constituted the French version of the social democracy that swept western Europe after the war, can be traced in large part to the turmoil of the 1930s. French leaders viewed the class conflict of that decade—its bitterly contested elections and violent strikes—as major factors in the nation's defeat at the hands of Germany in 1940.

As for ideology, these same leaders could not help but view laissez-faire capitalism with a deep distrust. Markets had crumbled around them during the Depression, leading to a downward spiral of economic despair that proved resistant to recovery by classic means. The resulting unemployment crisis and fall in living standards exacerbated the class conflicts of the 1930s. Plainly, market-based solutions had provided insufficient guarantees of economic stability. Under these conditions, it is hardly surprising that Resistance planners embraced forceful government action to promote health security for all after the war. In other words, Resistance planners viewed their charge as nothing less than to immunize France against renewed domestic strife and civil war.[6]

A further encouragement, if one were needed, came from the United States and Great Britain. Roosevelt's famous speech to Congress in January 1941, when he called for "freedom from want" for all citizens, proved far more inspiring to the French Resistance than to U.S. lawmakers, many of whom were by then in open revolt against New Deal social programs.[7] Resistance planners also looked to the British, in whose midst they lived, for an indication of whether grand social reform should precede or follow the return of economic prosperity. In 1942, William Beveridge released his plan for Britain's postwar welfare state, including the National Health Service. Shortly afterward, France's Resistance planners analyzed British public opinion and came to believe that, "for them [the British], the Beveridge Plan is an act of faith while at the same time it serves as a gauge of national and universal prosperity. That's why they will follow Beveridge who, when he is asked if the country has the means to undertake his plan, responds that the country does not have the wherewithal not to adopt it."[8]

British opinion of Beveridge's expansive social welfare plans emboldened Laroque; he came to believe that the most opportune moment for launching major reforms would be during the first year after Liberation. One planner even quoted Beveridge, exclaiming that "a revolutionary moment in the world's history is a time for revolution, not for patching."[9] But it was hardly a revolution that Resistance leaders wanted. Their intelligence operatives reported that the populace desired a "strong Republic" capable of offering "order, justice, and work."[10] De Gaulle hailed from the center-right of French politics, and Laroque stood just to the left of center. De Gaulle's legitimacy with Churchill and Roosevelt was always strained and stemmed in large measure from his ability to dominate a broad Resistance coalition whose effectiveness in skirmishes with Vichy and German forces increased steadily during the course of the war. From the Communist Left to the Christian Right, Resistance leaders agreed that a postliberation government would require broad powers of social and economic planning, a so-called *dirigiste* state, to rebuild a war-shaken nation. This, they believed, would be the best antidote for the humiliating defeat of 1940.[11]

Health Care under Sécurité Sociale

Once back in Paris, Pierre Laroque assumed leadership of the newly created *Sécurité Sociale* in early 1945. Although technically under Minister of Labor Alexandre Parodi, Laroque enjoyed great freedom of action because of his rapport with de Gaulle and other members of the Provisional Government. During the first months after Liberation, Laroque reported a strong esprit de corps among his staff as they set about preparing a comprehensive system of social welfare. Laroque's intimate involvement with the compromises and shortcomings of interwar and Vichy social protections clearly informed the audacious reforms that launched the country's postwar system of social protections.

Laroque professed three goals for *Sécurité Sociale*: administrative unity, national solidarity, and democratization. Although he failed to achieve the degree of administrative unity he had hoped for, Laroque nevertheless succeeded in creating a single institution for the governance of health, maternity, accident, disability, and retirement programs.[12] As a result of effective lobbying from natalist and familial groups, family allowance funds remained apart. Laroque's second principle, national solidarity, was to be achieved through the eventual extension of *Sécurité Sociale* to all citizens, including the self-employed, professionals, and managers. As under the 1930 social insurance law, payroll taxes provided the necessary revenue. Total premiums for social insurance rose to 16 percent of payroll. Of this total, employers paid 10 percent; the remaining 6 percent was withheld from workers' paychecks.

Laroque's last principle, democratization, stipulated that social insurance funds should be managed by beneficiaries, which, in short order, came to mean workers' unions. Although a few prominent employers, such as Marcel Michelin, emerged from the war with a list of patriotic feats to their credit, many more industrialists, including Louis Renault, had openly collaborated with the Nazi occupiers. As one Resistance document put it, "Some employers conducted themselves admirably. But collectively, employers were absent from the Resistance. . . . The government should replace the defunct employer confederation and take charge of purging the governing boards of employer associations."[13]

When administrative power over health insurance was handed over to *Sécurité Sociale*, mutual societies lost their intermediary role as insurance carriers. Mutual leaders responded by charging that "the government of national liberation [proposes] a plan . . . whose consequence is the suppression of one of the citizen's most fundamental liberties . . . that of free association." The national mutual society federation launched a massive effort to rally beneficiaries against *Sécurité Sociale*. They distributed thousands of posters and handbills, accusing the government of "wanting to institute in each department a system of cold and bureaucratic agencies into which beneficiaries will be integrated pell-mell, without their consent." Mutual leaders further warned that the creation of *Sécurité Sociale* would be "a brutal transformation" that would "rashly provoke a catastrophic disorganization whose victims will be social insurees."[14]

Despite the real dangers surrounding massive reform, mutual leaders' warnings fell on deaf ears, both within ruling circles and among the populace.[15] Not only had their image been tarnished by their association with the wartime Vichy regime; many regarded the social welfare of the 1930s inadequate for the new era. While Laroque never called into question the status of mutual societies as humanitarian civil society organizations, he noted that "mutual leaders most often belong to professional, management, and executive classes from industry and commerce and rarely to the wage-earning workers." Thus, as helpful as mutual leaders had been in administering the 1930 social insurance law, Laroque deemed their postwar insistence on continuing as privileged health care administrators out of step with France's newly enlarged sense of national solidarity. For Laroque, democratization meant that the "chief administrative officers of funds should come, for the most part, from the beneficiaries."[16]

Hence, the country's leading workers' union, the leftist CGT, became the heir apparent to most regional funds and the national board of *Sécurité Sociale*. In 1946, elections to the nation's 124 regional *Sécurité Sociale* boards resulted in 109 CGT majorities.[17] The predominance of CGT representatives on regional boards notwithstanding, *Sécurité Sociale* embraced the notion that welfare protections should be jointly managed by "social partners." The CGT could win a majority of seats on governing boards, but employers and mutual leaders were also guaranteed seats at the table, as were government officials. Although doctors were not granted a direct governing role in *Sécurité Sociale*, their representatives became critically important to its function. To express themselves, doctors quickly reconstituted the Confédération des Syndicats Médicaux Français (CSMF), which had been banned by the Vichy government during the war.

CSMF leaders promptly announced their objective to assert the principles of private practice in defense of "French medicine and doctors"; which, they promised, would have "a long and fruitful collaboration with public authorities" if they were respected.[18] Thus, no sooner had their first meeting been adjourned than doctors threw down the gauntlet to the gathering forces of *Sécurité Sociale*, headed by Laroque and backed by workers' unions. Laroque had been a keen observer of the failings of the 1930 health insurance law, especially its inability to adequately reimburse patients for doctors' fees. He therefore crafted what appeared to be a failsafe process to protect patients from high out-of-pocket costs.

Local medical *syndicats* were to propose a basic fee schedule, which would become part of a formal contract between local doctors and the departmental *Sécurité Sociale* board. A national board, a third of whose seats would be allocated to physicians, would in turn approve all departmental contracts. Doctors were permitted to exceed contractually defined fees when they rendered services under particularly difficult circumstances or by virtue of their renown. Under Laroque's plan, however, anyone could challenge a physician to justify his or her excess fees before a local panel consisting of two doctors and two *Sécurité Sociale* officials, one of whom had to be a physician.[19]

What is important here is that, despite the debacle of patient reimbursement in the 1930s, Laroque went to great lengths to preserve private fee-for-service medicine even when a historic opportunity might well have permitted a fundamental reform of French health care. Laroque never contemplated capitated payment schemes or a national health service, which was then being created in Great Britain. Under *Sécurité Sociale,* most French doctors remained private practitioners with unlimited clinical freedoms; medical confidentiality continued unchallenged; and the growing number of beneficiaries continued to enjoy direct access to general practitioners and specialists of their choosing. Moreover, French doctors, in contrast to their counterparts in much of the rest of Europe, continued to reject payment from third-party payers. Just as before the war, patients had to pay their doctors' bills and then seek reimbursement from *Sécurité Sociale*. Thus, despite the nation's embrace of solidarity and social equality, liberty and freedom of choice persisted as fundamental ideals in health care and medical practice.

With private medicine reanointed, this time with even more citizens paying into *Sécurité Sociale*, the old bugaboo of patient reimbursement re-emerged with a vengeance. Laroque's supposedly fail-safe process to ensure patient reimbursement at 80 percent of fees quickly fell by the wayside in the country's metropolitan centers. Local medical *syndicats* insisted on raising fees to keep up with the growing demand and the rising costs of delivering medical services. When regional *Sécurité Sociale* boards balked at raising their reimbursement rates so quickly, patients were again left holding the bill.

These difficulties, however, did not stand in the way of an unprecedented explosion in health care spending. In 1945, *Sécurité Sociale* extended ambulatory and hospital care, dental services, prescription drug coverage, wage loss stipends, and therapeutic hot springs visits to nearly half the population. By 1960, benefits had reached 76 percent of the populace, 31 percent of whom also enjoyed supplemental coverage, typically from mutual societies that picked up the tab for services that *Sécurité Sociale* failed to reimburse. The massive expansion in the demand for and supply of health care was hardly unique to France. Across Europe and the United States, a transformation of health and medical care was under way.

A New Definition of Health and the Explosion of Medical Care Costs

Theories abound to explain the postwar surge in health care prices and spending. Whatever their emphasis, observers agree that the phenomenon was multifaceted, with economic, political, and cultural causes being played out on both sides of the Atlantic.[20] To be sure, renewed economic prosperity and the spread of insurance played major roles. But they worked in tandem with a transformation in the definition of health and the nature of medical care. As medicine became increasingly efficacious in the treatment of what had previously been regarded as chronic or untreatable conditions, patients adopted a new attitude toward medical care. They no longer sought out their doctors only when poor health kept them from work or the routines of daily living. Now patients sought medical services to improve the quality of their lives. They wanted more than to merely restore bodily functions adversely affected by malady; they wanted better bodies. In other words, health was no longer simply the absence of illness, but rather, as the World Health Organization first put it in 1946, "a state of complete physical, mental and social well-being."[21]

In France, a 1960 poll found that 96 percent of the respondents viewed preventive medical care visits "indispensable" to their daily lives, an astounding increase from the interwar years, when few people sought medical services unless stricken by illness or accident.[22] Americans exhibited a similar newfound enthusiasm for health care. Between 1931 and the early 1950s, the proportion of the population that visited a doctor at least once a year rose from 48 to 72 percent. U.S. hospital admissions climbed 58 percent between 1945 and 1960. Sociological studies in both the United States and France in the 1950s found a marked increase in the citizenry's regard for medical services and in their willingness to purchase them.[23]

The increased use of hospitals led to a large hike in health care spending in both nations. Adjusted for inflation, French health care spending increased 129 percent between 1950 and 1958. The largest jump came in hospital services, which rose from 22.7 percent to 34.6 percent of total health care expenditures between 1947 and 1958.[24] France could afford the greatly increased outlays only by spending the surpluses accumulating in its retirement and family allowance funds. The United States experienced a similar surge in spending and there too hospital costs led the way. Between 1950 and 1965, per capita spending on U.S. community hospitals rose at the rate of 8 percent annually; after 1965, it increased 14 percent a year.[25] Moreover, in both countries, as more patients were admitted to hospitals in search of state-of-the-art surgical and curative care, the era of hospitals as hostels for the chronically ill and destitute came to a close. With their high expectations, the new patients demanded sanitary conditions and high-quality professional treatment that could only be delivered through the allocation of more resources. And the resources were readily available.

Blue Cross and *Sécurité Sociale* paid hospitals on the basis of their costs, a system under which hospitals had few incentives to increase efficiency. In fact, during the postwar hospital building boom, hospital administrators had every incentive to increase use, even if it meant needlessly extending patient stays. Empty beds meant lost revenue, pure and simple. According to a 1961 study, "When a hospital is under severe economic pressure to keep up the occupancy rate, it lacks the financial incentive to regulate admissions, or to press for shorter stays, or to tighten discharge procedure.... [An administrator would] try, consciously or unconsciously, to maintain in his institution the highest possible occupancy."[26]

Pharmaceuticals were also a major source of increased outlays. After hospitals, pharmaceutical spending presented the next largest increase for *Sécurité Sociale*, rising from 14.8 percent to 22.3 percent of total health care expenditures between 1947 and 1958.[27] Both nations embraced childhood vaccinations, enacting compulsory measures rather than permitting voluntary adherence. As a result, a battery of diseases that had once plagued young lives essentially disappeared. French leaders faced a century-old popular resentment against mandatory medical treatments of any kind, leading them to shy away from obligatory protections against less serious ailments, such as chicken pox. But they insisted that all schoolchildren be vaccinated against—not just tested for—tuberculosis. Immunizations and vaccinations, in and of themselves, were not expensive, but they brought a sharp fall in childhood mortality rates and a large rise in life expectancy. Eventually, these improvements greatly increased the prevalence of chronic diseases that occur later in life and are more expensive to treat.[28]

The growing prevalence of third-party payers also played a role in rising health care expenditures, since it encouraged patients to seek care that they believed had already been paid for through wage deductions, employer contributions, or other insurance premiums. And when they arrived for their appointments, they met physicians whose financial incentives encouraged them to practice more, not less, medicine. In France, doctors' *Sécurité Sociale* fee schedules were annually redrawn throughout the 1950s and virtually always contained substantial price hikes. Regional *Sécurité Sociale* boards usually contested those hikes, but patients were the ones who suffered in the event of dispute. U.S. practitioners also had wide discretion on how much their patients had to pay out of their own pockets. Under Blue Shield plans, physicians were somehow supposed to determine a patient's family income when preparing the bill, because many plans provided comprehensive medical services (not just an indemnity) for those whose income fell below a contractual threshold. Depending on the doctor's decision, the patient's out-of-pocket expenses ranged from zero to as much as half the bill.[29] In the final analysis, French physicians' power over fees (both collectively and individually) resembled U.S. doctors' insistence that insurers respect what the 1965 Medicare legislation would eventually label "usual, customary, and reasonable" charges.

To define what was "customary and reasonable," doctors in both countries did not just look at the underlying inflation of their inputs, that is, the cost of wages, rent, bandages, and so forth. They also inevitably took note of what their colleagues were charging. After the war, when the demand for medical care was rising and many new doctors were opening up practices, "usual and customary" billing led inexorably to rampant fee increases that bore scant relation to the general inflation indexes and even exceeded the greater price rises of medical equipment and training. The sociologist Paul Starr captures the dynamic in the United States: "Fees began to soar when some young doctors, who had no record of charges, billed at unprecedented levels and were paid [by insurers]. When their older colleagues saw what was possible, they, too, raised their fees, and soon what was customary was higher than ever before."[30] Or, as one *Sécurité Sociale* official observed, fee increases "that are accepted quickly become trampolines for doctors elsewhere who are also demanding increases."[31]

In U.S. and French cities, where the number of medical practices rose quickly in the 1950s, fees skyrocketed. This, of course, runs contrary to most other supply-and-demand scenarios, under which an increase in supply of a product translates into more competition between suppliers and lower prices for consumers. But because patients (consumers) were not paying the bill and doctors (suppliers) were in a position to counsel consumers to buy more at higher prices, costs rose. In addition, patients *wanted* to buy more medical care, not just because they were insulated from its cost but also because of health care's greater effectiveness and the higher standard of what constituted "good health."

It is hard to pinpoint the relative importance of the various causes behind health care price increases and spending during the immediate postwar decades. But it is clear that costs were forced up by a synergy between fantastic (but expensive) gains in the effectiveness of medicine, a new definition of health that spurred a stronger demand for health care, and fee-for-service medical practice that dictated that insurers stand clear of the doctor-patient relationship and exert only minimum surveillance over physicians' clinical and fee-setting authorities. No matter where the greater or lesser responsibility for health care inflation lay, workers responded angrily to the increased costs, which affected their take-home pay and benefits.

Common Struggles: Labor's Quest for Control of Health Care in France and the United States

One might suspect that France's labor unions would be in a far better position to influence health care delivery and to hold down costs than were their U.S. counterparts in the 1950s. After all, the powerful CGT, its offshoot, the CGT-FO, and the smaller Christian Democratic CFTC together dominated the regional and national governing boards of *Sécurité Sociale*. U.S. labor unions, meanwhile, including the mighty AFL and CIO, could negotiate with employers over health care benefits only at the collective bargaining table. In all but a small number of trades, U.S. labor leaders had no formal rights over the administration of health insurance funds. In fact, in the vast majority of cases, employers—not workers—enjoyed the legal status of contracting party with Blue Cross, Blue Shield, and commercial insurers.

Despite markedly different relations to their respective health care industries, however, French and U.S. union leaders experienced surprisingly similar frustrations in the late 1940s and 1950s. At root was health care's rapidly swelling price, which in both countries was being financed from wages. To be sure, employers also paid a hefty share. But as employers themselves so often insisted when bargaining with workers, management's share of health insurance premiums came out of potential cash wages, which employees forfeited when they demanded generous health benefits. Beginning in the 1950s, the large price hikes in hospital and ambulatory care were passed on to workers in the form of reduced reimbursements, increased premiums, reduced services, or all three. This motivated union leaders and employers in France and the United States to seek greater control over health care finance and delivery, a quest that ultimately led to a further divergence in the two nations' health care systems.

Soon after their election to *Sécurité Sociale* boards in 1946, France's labor leaders discovered that their status as privileged "social partners" gave them insufficient clout to meet the challenges that confronted them. To be sure, union officials controlled a massive purse—fully 16 percent of the wages of half the population then participating in *Sécurité Sociale*. They also possessed substantial administrative prerogatives over each of France's social insurance programs: health, disability, accident, family allowances, and retirement pensions. But lawmakers they were not.

When health care costs rose nearly twice as fast as wages, union leaders exercised the only two options available to them.[32] They redirected as much revenue as possible from other *Sécurité Sociale* programs, namely, family allowances and retirement funds, to cover the deficit. When these additional funds proved insufficient, *Sécurité Sociale* simply could not fulfill its commitment to reimburse patients 80 percent of doctors' fees, as patients had been promised in 1945.[33] Because health insurance premiums were set by law as a percentage of wages and not—as in the United States—at the collective bargaining table, *Sécurité Sociale* leaders looked first to the medical profession for help. What they found frustrated them.

Especially in France's largest cities, including Paris, Lyons, and Marseilles, local medical leaders rejected on philosophical grounds the idea that patients could be assured any particular level of reimbursement. As one medical leader put it, "Reimbursement at a fixed rate obviously presupposes that fees are set in advance, somehow 'scheduled.'... Doctors have always viewed this and continue to view this as an attack on our professional freedoms."[34] To the great consternation of *Sécurité Sociale* officials, this view persisted even in departments where medical leaders had signed contracts that included fee schedules. Doctors insisted that no advance agreement on fees could ultimately prevent an individual practitioner from charging what he or she thought appropriate. To hold otherwise, they believed, would be a violation of their professional sovereignty.

This position resulted in many tense negotiations between *Sécurité Sociale* boards and doctors, at both the departmental and national levels. On one occasion, the usually reserved executive director of the national *Sécurité Sociale* board, Clément Michel, became exasperated when his physician interlocutors kept insisting that, even though they had freely agreed to a fee schedule, any expectations that they would abide by it was, in their words, "imposing doctors' fees." "Doctors' absolute liberty makes it impossible," Michel observed, "for us to achieve an 80 percent reimbursement [of our beneficiaries]. If there is no contract, no agreement, there will be nothing but a fee to which you are only ethically bound." Exactly, replied the doctors: "A third party placed [between the patient and his doctor], in addition to the abuse and demoralization that it engenders, destroys the patient's sense of personal responsibility. It debases the dignity of man."[35] Hence, according to doctors, the principles of private-practice medicine trumped any statutes, legal contracts, or social responsibility that might intrude on physicians' liberty of medical practice, which included the right to set fees.

U.S. physicians were also unwilling to abide by predetermined fee schedules. In Ohio, the United Rubber Workers thought they had reached an agreement with doctors to "follow closely a schedule of payments," only to learn that, as in the French case, the agreement meant little to individual practitioners. A contract with the Los Angeles County Medical Association met a similar fate. In San Francisco, the California Metal Trades Association and the Labor Council negotiated for two years in an attempt to reach an accord with the local medical society. The only result was a schedule of exorbitant fees, to which the medical society added the statement: "No member of the Society is obligated to work by this schedule." According to the historian Raymond Munts, San Francisco doctors typified the U.S. medical profession's lack of regard for negotiations over fees. In a comment that might have been lifted word for word from a French counterpart, a San Francisco medical leader insisted, "There must be no set or frozen fee schedule.... The doctor's right to establish with his patient the fee to be paid must be respected.... There can be no 'third party' placed in the middle of the all-important and confidential doctor-patient relationship."[36]

In France, labor leaders who administered *Sécurité Sociale* resolved to obtain more money from the government to ensure proper reimbursement of beneficiaries. In 1953 they signed an accord that instructed regional *Sécurité Sociale* boards to conclude contracts that would provide practitioners most of what they wanted. With contracts in place, labor leaders thought, the government would be forced to meet their contractual obligations, even if it meant digging into the government treasury. Instead, political leaders balked, citing the cost of France's protracted war in Algeria. The French government's refusal to assure adequate funding for patient reimbursement indicated that a much larger issue was at stake than just a disagreement over priorities between *Sécurité Sociale* and government ministers. Health care's tie to employment had once again emerged as a structural flaw that undermined equity and access to the nation's growing medical services.

In both countries, wages provided a major revenue source for the rapidly expanding health care infrastructure of hospital and ambulatory care services. Also in both nations, despite the heavy reliance on paycheck deductions and employer contributions, neither the workers nor the employers who paid insurance premiums enjoyed any substantial compensatory control over health care delivery. By the early 1950s, France's *Sécurité Sociale* board had recognized its impotence vis-à-vis doctors and the government, admitting that "the sovereignty of *Sécurité Sociale* boards is more nominal than real."[37] The board added that "the financing of *Sécurité Sociale* is profoundly unjust. The law not only demands that wage earners finance their own benefits through a redistribution of income but also that they pay for the hospital and antitubercular infrastructure, as well as for the administration of the labor ministry."[38] Secretly, French government officials agreed. In a confidential memo, the director of *Sécurité Sociale*, Pierre Laroque, bluntly reported that "it is possible to say, without exaggeration, that the quasi-totality of the population ... realizes substantial material benefits from [the health insurance system] ... while the only ones who are regular contributors are...the permanent wage earners." This unseemly situation had arisen because, after the initial burst of expansion of *Sécurité Sociale* between 1945 and 1947, some sectors of the labor force had blocked their incorporation into it.

When the Communist minister of labor, Ambroise Croizat, called for the universalization of *Sécurité Sociale* in 1947, conservative and centrist political leaders took up the cause of the salaried middle class and the self-employed. They opposed their inclusion in *Sécurité Sociale* on pointedly parochial grounds, arguing that their enrollment was a financing ploy pure and simple, meant to subsidize lower premiums for the working class.[39] Yet, having prevailed in blocking expansion and thereby their obligation to pay premiums, many self-employed and salaried professionals nonetheless gained access to *Sécurité Sociale* services when they so desired. Something called "adverse selection" had become a major threat to *Sécurité Sociale*.

In his memo, Laroque devoted considerable attention to the problem of adverse selection, an insurance industry term that describes conditions under which risks not contemplated by the insurer nevertheless become insured. For example, Laroque bemoaned at length the case of a self-employed business owner—one outside *Sécurité Sociale,* therefore—whose fourteen-year-old son required expensive surgery. The businessman simply found another small business owner to "hire" his son as an hourly wage earner for a few weeks so that the surgery would be entirely paid for, minus a few weeks' premiums, by *Sécurité Sociale*. Although frustrated by the fraud, Laroque clearly understood that to deny that such "false wage earners" needed medical treatment would prove extremely difficult, perhaps even impossible, given the wall of doctor-patient confidentiality and the ease of access to medical care that all "real wage earners" rightfully expected. Laroque continued, "We are confronted with the paradox that our health insurance system rests on limited solidarity among wage earners, who are in general of the most modest means, but that a number of salaried and self-employed workers regularly take advantage of them." For Laroque, of course, the paradox could be most effectively resolved by "extending compulsory health insurance to the entire population, [which] would reestablish equity between those who pay and those who benefit."[40]

Perhaps because they were sometimes complicit, doctors also seemed aware of the adverse selection problem that afflicted *Sécurité Sociale*. They opposed universalization on principle, warning that it would mark a further move toward a British-style national health service and therewith the destruction of private-practice fee-for-service medicine. But they shared labor leaders' frustration that payroll taxes alone could not possibly pay for the vast health care use and price increases. Quite in their own interest, then, doctors noted that, "if *Sécurité Sociale* must apply to everyone…then it is obvious that the system of wage-based premiums must be abandoned and replaced by a general health tax."[41]

If change must come, French doctors reasoned, they wanted to gain access to the government treasury, which would both alleviate their bitter relations with the labor leaders who ran *Sécurité Sociale* boards and end the gallingly low reimbursements suffered by their patients. In short, "usual, customary, and reasonable" fees would become all the more upwardly mobile. This same logic would eventually bring U.S. doctors to embrace Medicare, for it too made the U.S. Treasury liable for rapidly rising medical fees. Well before that, however, U.S. labor leaders had made their own bid to assume meaningful control over health care.

By 1954, 12 million workers and 17 million of their dependents enjoyed collectively bargained health benefits. Such plans help explain how 60 percent of the U.S. population had gained some form of health insurance by 1954.[42] Yet like French labor's frustration with *Sécurité Sociale,* U.S. union leaders soon realized that their victories at the bargaining table were only half the battle. What they really needed was influence over the workings of health care finance and delivery itself. Otherwise, the dramatic price rises in hospital and ambulatory care would take ever-larger slices of their paychecks.[43]

U.S. labor unions generally preferred Blue Cross, and to a lesser extent, Blue Shield, during the immediate postwar war decades. This preference stemmed not only from the Blues' avowedly community service orientation and nonprofit status, but also from the perception among union leaders that commercial insurers were unscrupulous and in collusion with employers. Firms that purchased health insurance from commercial insurers were eligible for so-called dividends each year, depending on whether the insurer had met its profit margin over and above its costs for insuring company workers. Workers justifiably viewed these payments as wage-funded kickbacks to employers for selecting a commercial insurer.[44] Moreover, Blue Cross and Blue Shield offered exceptionally good medical and hospital service plans. Far from all physicians would accept payment from a third payer, but those who did almost always dealt with Blue Shield because of its official recognition by the AMA. Most hospitals were similarly committed to Blue Cross plans, whose governing boards included hospital administrators.

As the price and utilization of hospital and medical services rose dramatically in the 1950s, U.S. labor leaders sought what French labor leaders had won in 1945: seats on the governing boards of health care insurers. New York provides an exemplary case of what happened when U.S. unions went after a formal role in the administration of Blue Cross.

The Battle for Health Insurer Boardrooms

The contest between New York labor unions and Blue Cross erupted in 1957 when the hospital service plan announced a 40 percent increase in premiums. The previous year, local United Auto Workers' leaders had warned that Blue Cross seemed bent on maintaining cash reserves well above legal minimums and that board members were insufficiently attentive to holding down hospital costs. After the announcement of the premium hike, other unions joined in the criticism of Blue Cross, prompting a citywide debate about the nature and role of Blue Cross in the community. Walter Eisenberg of the CIO Council insisted that Blue Cross had abandoned its "fundamental idea" as "a joint user and supplier vehicle for the provision of pre-paid hospital service." He charged that Blue Cross had become a "producer's cooperative run for the primary purpose of stabilizing an ever-larger portion of the income of the suppliers, that is, the hospitals." Eisenberg recommended that labor organizations be granted 50 percent of Blue Cross board seats.[45]

This idea sounded reasonable to the editors of the *New York Times*. They opined that Blue Cross had "not given its subscribers and the public the status they should have—especially in dealing with the hospitals as to charges." In a subsequent editorial, the *Times* backed a United Steel Workers economist who called upon Blue Cross to "be directed away from the singled minded concern with meeting unquestionably every demand of the hospitals and toward a balanced view which impartially gives equal weight to the needs of hospitals, subscribers and the public interest."[46]

Fearful about its relationship with organized labor, Blue Cross announced no additional premium hikes throughout 1958; and when four board seats opened up, it filled three with labor representatives. Yet this concession only provoked hospital leaders to demonstrate the hard truth to labor unions about who really controlled Blue Cross, and health care more generally. The United Hospital Fund, which included sixty-six hospitals in the greater New York area, exercised its until-then unused statutory right to create and appoint seven entirely new seats, thereby swamping any greater influence over Blue Cross policies that unions might have gained with their three board members.

The desire to remain firmly in control of hospital care finance and delivery was not the only thing behind the United Hospital Fund's maneuver. By the mid-1950s, hospitals and their associated medical complexes had become technologically sophisticated and potentially lucrative profit centers in a growing health care industry. This transformation was not lost on New York unions, especially since the booming hospitals employed large numbers of low-paid, unorganized workers. Just as union officials and sympathetic political activists launched their criticism of Blue Cross's premium increases, a new local was being created for hospital workers. In the spring of 1959, thirty-five hundred members of Local 1199 launched a forty-six-day strike at hospitals across the city. Although some union leaders viewed the strike as more hurtful to patients than to hospitals, many more publicly contrasted Blue Cross's "excessive and unjustified" premium increases with the low wages still being paid to hospital workers. The only explanation, labor leaders concluded, was that Blue Cross had become "little more than a collection agency for hospitals."[47] Hospital administrators, conversely, felt besieged on two fronts—first in the Blue Cross boardroom and now on the picket line. Naturally, they met labor's thrust with a forceful riposte.

Meanwhile, the bloom was also off the rose in labor's relationship with Blue Shield. Unions had embraced the AMA-sanctioned plans during the war for many of the same reasons that they preferred Blue Cross: Blue Shield's not-for-profit mission and its service benefits. Yet in 1954 a study by a New Jersey Blue Shield official, James Bryan, found that too many plans around the country had instituted substantial restrictions on comprehensive coverage, thereby imitating "the worst commercial insurance company practices." Bryan's report revealed that thirty Blue Shield plans limited their surgical benefits to two hundred dollars, which, even in the 1950s, represented an insufficient contribution for many procedures.

In 1957, United Steel Workers spokesperson John Tomayko complained to an audience of Blue Shield leaders that "Blue Shield alone held out the possibility to us that through its official relations with physicians it could provide a means whereby the surgical and other costly medical bills could be paid in full.... [Now] the Steelworkers believe that Blue Shield has lost sight of its original purpose and has deteriorated into a collection agency for the medical profession." For his candor, Tomayko received a chorus of hisses and boos from the assembled Blue Shield officials.[48] They justifiably believed that Blue Shield plans remained the workers' best choice for physician services insurance. But for labor leaders, who watched helplessly as doctors' fees steadily rose year after year, "best choice" had a bitter ring. U.S. labor was then approaching its zenith of political and economic might in the twentieth century. But at the very same moment, the greatest unions in the country appeared powerless to affect the course of an increasingly large portion of workers' compensation.

When all was said and done, an unlikely parallel existed between the plight of U.S. labor leaders and their French counterparts as they confronted rising health care costs in the 1950s. Even though French unions had boardroom majorities, the insurer that they controlled, *Sécurité Sociale*, could, by itself, neither hold down medical costs nor raise premiums. Meanwhile, the AFL had only token representation on Blue Cross's more powerful boards and none on Blue Shield, both of which had considerable influence over costs and premiums. Yet for French and U.S. unions, the net effect was the same. Labor leaders in both countries felt deprived of what they deemed to be their due influence over the health security of their members, who, after all, provided a major share of the health care industry's revenue.

Not surprisingly then, U.S. and French unions pursued comparable strategies, which they hoped would improve their influence over medical care providers. Their first hope was for labor to build its own health care system. In France, all unions openly endorsed the advantages of *Sécurité Sociale*–run pharmacies and clinics as well as a state-directed health service to staff them.[49] In New York, where unions were battling hospitals for Blue Cross board seats, it was an open secret that labor leaders were studying the feasibility of using monies from their pension funds to build and operate their own hospitals. Indeed, a wave of union interest in "labor health centers" swept the United States in the mid-1950s. Union officials in New York, Philadelphia, Washington, D.C., Saint Louis, and San Francisco succeeded in building clinics of varying sizes, which quickly became models for other unions.

The grandfather of union-run health care had been created by the United Mine Workers in the late 1940s. Their leader, John Lewis, led an epic strike in 1947–1948, eventually forcing the Truman administration to take over the mines. Having provoked federal intervention from a government that favored national health insurance, Lewis held the upper hand when he demanded that mine owners fully fund an array of clinics and hospitals, which the mine workers' union would administer as an equal partner.[50] But the mine workers' health care system proved impossible to replicate elsewhere because of its unique origins and employer financing.

Unions in France and the United States also attempted to create networks of medical providers, that is, physicians, hospitals, and allied health professionals who agreed to treat their members under predetermined payment arrangements. Soon after it became apparent that French medical *syndicats* were unwilling to curtail individual practitioners' freedom to set fees, a CGT representative on the national *Sécurité Sociale* board suggested that regional boards "identify doctors who will accept the normal *Sécurité Sociale* fees and to circulate their names [among social insurees]."[51] U.S. union leaders were equally active in this regard, especially those in the building trades. Using this strategy, unions bypassed medical societies altogether to obtain predictable prices. In both nations, these tactics ultimately proved inadequate (and difficult for us to trace) because participating physicians preferred that the lists be kept confidential by workers' organizations.

In response, medical leaders used their considerable influence to scare off practitioners who might otherwise have signed on to union lists. In 1956, the Painters' Fund in the San Francisco Bay Area—ten thousand members strong—created probably the most successful union network, but with only forty-three doctors it had little practical effect in helping members avoid the unpleasant surprise of high out-of-pocket charges.[52] Although unions ultimately failed to cobble together enough practitioners to create workable networks, many succeeded in holding down medical costs by turning to group practices.

In France, this meant mutual societies, which since the 1930s had been a locus for practitioners, especially surgeons, who were willing to accept set salaries in exchange for a guaranteed clientele and technologically sophisticated practice conditions. After the war, despite having lost the prominent role they had played under the first compulsory health insurance law of 1930, mutual societies experienced a renaissance. The salaried and self-employed middle classes, who had not yet been enrolled in *Sécurité Sociale*, sought out mutual societies in large numbers, both through employer group plans and individual policies. Also, as patient reimbursements from *Sécurité Sociale* failed to keep pace with rising medical fees, mutual societies found many in the working class who were eager to purchase supplemental health insurance, especially for costly surgical procedures. Mutual societies provided employers and workers with reassuring promises of full-service medical care at predictable prices, something that doctors in private practice, backed by their medical *syndicats*, were unwilling to provide.[53] By 1958, one in twenty French citizens underwent surgery of some kind. The average cost for a procedure was fifty thousand francs, or about four hundred (1958) dollars. Alongside its increased effectiveness, supplemental mutual society insurance played a large role in the swelling demand for surgery. By 1958, French mutual societies boasted 8.5 million subscribers and a growth rate of 12 percent a year.[54] In the United States, workers and employers opted for group practice plans for reasons similar to those that led their French counterparts to purchase supplemental mutual insurance: to escape the unpredictable and rising prices of fee-for-service medicine.

Kaiser Health Plans were among the most successful. Kaiser had begun as a paternalist employer program, when the concrete magnate Henry Kaiser won large public works programs throughout the West in the 1930s. Wartime production led to a further expansion of Kaiser's industrial enterprises, especially in shipbuilding. After the war, he opened his hospitals and clinics to the public for prepaid group and individual enrollment. By 1956, Kaiser had attracted just over half a million members and harbored ambitious plans for a national expansion.

Yet Kaiser possessed neither a long history of health care provision nor the credentials of a civil society organization. In other words, for all its efficiency and quality, Kaiser lacked the popular legitimacy that was a crucial ingredient to the public embrace of Blue Cross plans before the war. This newcomer status notwithstanding, Kaiser presented a reassuring and fresh vision of health security. Similar to his innovations in concrete and shipbuilding, Kaiser hoped to create the "new economies of medicine."[55] And to a great extent, he succeeded. Where Kaiser plans were available on the West Coast, union workers often preferred them to commercial plans and even the Blues. A 1960 United Steel Workers study found that while union members reported little difference between hospital coverage across plans, they reported much greater satisfaction with Kaiser physician services.[56]

What astonished the steel workers' leadership (and troubled medical leaders) was that Kaiser's most blatant violations of private-practice medicine occurred in physician services, the very area where workers expressed most satisfaction. An emotional 1953 confrontation in Pittsburgh, California, between Kaiser and the local medical society provided further evidence that some workers prized assurance of nearly full coverage over choice of private-practice physician. When Kaiser opened a new hospital in the nearby community of Walnut Creek, local doctors launched a massive campaign to convince the four thousand members of United Steel Workers

Local 1440 that a local doctor's plan would provide better care and service at virtually the same price. The physicians' campaign included full-page newspaper ads, leaflets, a sound truck, and direct appeals to workers between shifts in the plant parking lot by doctors' family members.

The doctors' slogans came straight from the principles of private-practice medicine and could have been used by French physicians against their mutual society rivals: "Retain your family doctor"; "Don't be a captive patient." On polling day, the steelworkers voted overwhelmingly for Kaiser (2,182 to 440). Clearly, the steelworkers had doubted the genuineness of the doctor's plan. Indeed, after the vote, the plan disappeared, even though the medical society had promised it would be available to other members of the community.[57] Although Kaiser presented an appealing option for some West Coast populations, it never realized its hopes for an eastward expansion. Its battles with fee-for-service medical practitioners, however, offered a glimpse of U.S. workers, who would embrace group practices, known as HMOs, later in the century.

In fact, the vitality of Kaiser in the West, the resurgence of French mutual societies, and the ongoing struggle among labor unions, insurers, and health care providers, showed that the hallowed principles of private-practice medicine were not as invulnerable as they had once seemed. As medical costs continued to rise and larger portions of the population gained access to health insurance, workers sought broad assurances of comprehensive health security and demonstrated their willingness to sacrifice physician choice to obtain it.

No doubt, the new definition of health that began to take hold after the Second World War affected this pursuit of health security. Thereafter, a growing attentiveness to "good health" paradoxically made its attainment all the more difficult. New medical science techniques meant more effective diagnoses and therapies, which in turn spurred greater demand for medicine, leading to still more spending to obtain even better medicine. Thus, in contrast to its interwar definition, good health had become like the horizon: the faster one ran toward it, the more quickly it receded out of reach. The pursuit of health translated into incredible gains in life expectancy and physical quality of life for millions in France and the United States. But as the cost of health care continued its skyward direction, it provoked diverse responses from U.S. and French political leaders.

6

THE CHOICE OF PUBLIC OR PRIVATE, 1950–1970

I saved France on a colonel's pay. For the billions I pay you, surely you can give me better health care!

PRESIDENT CHARLES DE GAULLE, addressing physicians in 1960

A 1951 tour by French medical leaders of the United States provides us with a telling glimpse into the different choices that each nation made between public and private insurance. The French doctors stopped first in New York, where they met George Baehr, medical director of the Health Insurance Plan of Greater New York, a group practice founded by Mayor Fiorello LaGuardia. The plan offered prepaid medical services to city employees and later spread to include three hundred thousand subscribers in and around greater New York. Baehr was LaGuardia's personal physician and had been instrumental in the plan's creation. The New York plan complemented Blue Cross (for hospitalization), but it competed fiercely with New York's Blue Shield, which offered insurance for physician services under the standard precepts of fee-for-service private practice.

To his French visitors, Baehr constantly emphasized the advantages of group practice: generalist and specialist collaboration, quality and cost assurance for patients, and, given the large number of doctors in the New York plan, substantial patient choice of physician. The French doctors nevertheless registered unease about restrictions on a patient's choice and even more concern about the health plan's powerful role as a third-party payer between patient and doctor.

At their second stop, AMA headquarters in Chicago, the French doctors found themselves in better harmony with their interlocutors. Indeed, they appeared to enjoy the lively criticism of the New York group practice expressed by their AMA hosts. The French also got a little taste of the McCarthy era in the United States when one of the AMA officials gravely warned his guests about "the political beliefs that surround this sort of health insurance." Yet for all their agreement about patient choice and, no doubt, conservative politics, the French physicians were still disturbed by their U.S. counterpart's blithe embrace of third-party payers, in both New York and Chicago.

It is clear from the French account of the trip that U.S. doctors were proud of the leading role physician-sanctioned Blue Shield plans were playing in the nation's growing private voluntary health insurance system. The French doctors were dazzled by their hosts' sophisticated knowledge of insurance and the "economic and actuarial aspects of medical practice." Yet as impressed as they were, the purist French held fast to their belief that any third party between the individual doctor and the patient from whom the doctor collected fees—even a third party ostensibly controlled by physicians—represented a mortal danger to the doctor-patient relationship. Equally telling, French physicians reported unease among their U.S. colleagues regarding the possibility of public health insurance in the United States. Their U.S. hosts insisted that such a development "threatened to alter the foundations of American civilization," a comment that clearly puzzled the French.[1]

When all was said and done, the French doctors viewed as contradictory their U.S. colleagues' lenient position on third-party payers on the one hand, and their extreme conservatism toward compulsory insurance on the other. How, wondered the French, could the Americans be so horrified by public health insurance but so complacent about taking money directly from insurers, a practice they viewed as a slippery slope toward losing control over medical decision making? Likewise, the Americans had to be perplexed by their guests' support of public health insurance even as the French forever swore off working directly with private insurers, who, from the U.S. point of view, offered the best way to protect medicine from government meddling.

This is not to say that U.S. physicians opposed all government intervention. They had readily endorsed a massive federal government appropriation bill for hospital construction, the Hill-Burton Act, whose outlays ranged between 75 and 186 million dollars each year between 1948 and 1961.[2] Nor is it to suggest that the U.S. and French doctors were uniform in their views on fee-for-service private practice. Many U.S. and French physicians alike were attracted to group practices such as Kaiser and mutual society clinics, whose postwar expansion reflected workers' frustration with rising health care bills, a frustration some physicians clearly shared.

In general, however, the medical profession in both nations was struggling to maintain the primacy of private-practice medicine in vastly different ways during an era of rapid changes in health care and their peoples' growing expectations for health security. Having embraced voluntary private health insurance to fend off legislative initiatives for national health insurance during the Roosevelt and Truman administrations, U.S. doctors were determined to maintain a leading role in its evolution, both by propagating Blue Shield plans and by continuing their legislative activism. In this regard, the AMA closely followed the advice of its California public relations consultants, Clem Whitaker and Leone Baxter, who told their clients, "If we can get ten million more people insured in the next year and ten million more in the next year, the threat of socialized medicine in this country will be over."[3] Many in the U.S. business community joined the AMA in its support of private health insurance. *Business Week* advised its readership that, if management failed to heed labor's call for health security, "the worker is likely to transfer his demands from the bargaining table to the ballot box."[4] Such advocacy and hopes for the growth of private third-party payers led inexorably to the AMA's abandonment of its long opposition to control of private health insurance by nonmedical personnel.[5]

The Tension between Interdependent Citizenship and Liberty

In the late 1940s and 1950s, both nations witnessed comparable struggles over what constituted the proper mix between interdependent citizenship and individual liberty. In France, the struggle became apparent when the self-employed and salaried middle-class professions blocked their own incorporation into *Sécurité Sociale* until the 1960s because they feared their contributions would serve merely to subsidize the health care expenses of others. In the United States, where private actors held considerably more power, the struggle over whether to pursue more interdependence in health care can be seen in the evolution of insurance pricing. At their inception, the Blues adopted "community rating," whereby all employer groups were thrown together into a single pool and risk was divided evenly among them by means of a single premium rate. Under "experience rating," conversely, insurers set premiums for each individual group based on its risk and actual loss experience.

By the mid-1960s, when the self-employed and the salaried middle classes finally embraced *Sécurité Sociale*, it became clear that France had opted for citizen interdependence in the pursuit of health security. Already in 1958, a poll of 3,910 randomly selected *Sécurité Sociale* beneficiaries from across France reflected remarkable support for sharing risk. Fully 95 percent of respondents said that the compulsory nature of health insurance was "a good thing." When pollsters asked: "Do you believe that everyone should get back what they paid into *Sécurité Sociale* or is it fair that the healthy pay for the sick?" just over 86 percent responded that "the healthy should pay for the sick." Fifty-four percent of respondents also indicated that they possessed supplemental mutual society health insurance to protect themselves from risks and costs not covered by *Sécurité Sociale*. Indeed, 62 percent of those polled complained that they received "a lot less than 80 percent" in reimbursements for their doctor's bills. Physician charges topped their list (at 41 percent) as the least adequately reimbursed medical expense. (Dental care came in second at 23 percent.)[6]

The United States, meanwhile, was drifting away from citizen interdependence for health security and toward more parochial solutions. A 1944 University of Denver poll found that a substantial proportion of Americans (58 percent) supported the expansion of Social Security to include compulsory health insurance.[7] Reflecting this postwar view, U.S. labor organizations consistently backed national health insurance. The AFL and the CIO pooled funds and expertise to form an umbrella group, the Committee on the Nation's Health, which lobbied Congress on behalf of Truman's postwar health insurance initiative.[8] These efforts by the unions, however, were inescapably tempered by their simultaneous pursuit of private health insurance at the collective bargaining table. Labor was also consistently outspent by the AMA—1.5 million to 104,000 dollars in 1949 alone.[9] Yet ambivalence among the rank and file, especially in the CIO, where 95 percent of members had employer-based private insurance by 1948, also dampened enthusiasm for national health insurance. Simply put, labor's Committee on the Nation's Health could not rely on mass mobilization to achieve its ends.[10]

Deprived of their best punches, union advocates for national health insurance pursued alliances with like-minded social reform groups within and outside labor. When Harry Truman, like his predecessor, Franklin Roosevelt, became increasingly reluctant to use the presidential bully pulpit to do anything more than urge in a general way for a national health policy, labor's campaign for national health insurance quickly grew unconvincing. In the words of one labor leader, "The benefits workers get under the [private] health . . . plans are so much better than those we have dared to include in the health insurance bills [in Congress] that it has become an anomaly for us to continue to favor compulsory health insurance."[11] After the election of the Republican Dwight Eisenhower to the presidency in 1956, Republicans asked the AMA to write their health care platform, a task that medical leaders enthusiastically accepted. The possibility, if not the issue, of national health insurance disappeared from the national agenda.[12]

By 1958, two-thirds of all Americans had some form of private health insurance coverage.[13] Much of this progress, however, was made possible by the spread of experience-rated rather than community-rated insurance. Because they had been blocked in their bid for formal control of insurers and medical care providers, U.S. unions and employers held down their health care premium hikes by working with insurers. Together they sectioned off their members and employees from other groups with relatively sicker and more accident-prone enrollees, and in so doing gained lower premiums and better benefits. A new law, the Taft-Hartley Act of 1947, proved critical to this development.

Taft-Hartley was payback, pure and simple, by the Republicans for the previous decade and a half, during which Democratic-controlled Congresses had coddled their union supporters. Its immediate motivation was a wave of strikes that swept the country after unions were freed of their no-strike pledge at the end of the Second World War. Although Republican lawmakers could not remove health insurance from the collective bargaining table, the Taft-Hartley Act greatly limited the operation of union health and retirement funds. Unions could no longer independently administer welfare benefits to which employers had contributed; they now had to follow Taft-Hartley's rules. But because the new law also prohibited closed shops, it actually encouraged unions to embrace the new Taft-Hartley–governed health and pension benefits all the more fervently.

Closed shops were worksites where union membership constituted a precondition for employment. Once they were prohibited, union leaders came to view union-won health and welfare benefits as a substitute means for building and sustaining worker loyalty to the union. Or, as the political scientist Michael Brown puts it, the Taft-Hartley welfare funds became "the virtual equivalent of a closed shop" because, in order to gain access to fund benefits, a worker had to join the union.[14] Taft-Hartley plans grew especially fast in unionized trades where members commonly worked for several firms over the course of a single year, such as in the building trades and seasonal industries. Within two years after passage, Taft-Hartley plans dispensed benefits to over 3 million workers and double that many dependents. Where they succeeded, the new funds placed labor leaders in a powerful bargaining position vis-à-vis commercial insurers and the Blues.[15]

Just as employers had earlier given in to the temptation of experience rating, union leaders now collaborated in its spread. Experience rating offered union health insurance funds an effective tool for carving out better benefits while minimizing premium increases. Insurers' underwriters told them that the risk of extending coverage to groups of workers was far less than that for the general population, where adverse selection and moral hazard presented greater dangers.

Once employers and labor leaders had tasted experience rating, their appetite for the policies grew apace with the insurance industry's sophistication at brewing them. Soon insurers developed an assortment of nuanced policies geared to different trades and professions, each with its own premiums, exclusions, and special provisions, based on the latest experience data. At first, the Blues responded with horror. In 1953, Blue Cross's national rating committee urged hospital plans around the country to eschew experience rating altogether. Five years later, only twenty-two of seventy-seven Blue Cross plans adhered to the advice. By 1967, only one community-rated Blue remained.[16] The competitive pressures from commercial insurers, egged on by demands from employers and labor leaders for the best coverage at the lowest possible price, were simply too great to resist.[17] Even Robert Taft, the Republican coauthor of the Taft-Hartley Act, warned that such important welfare benefits might ultimately need to be "integrated with social security" so that health care would "not be broken up into a series of industry agreements."[18] As the addiction to experience rating grew, it acquired powerful constituencies in the middle and working classes, groups that might have provided a core of support for national health insurance. Now even the most conservative legislators came to realize that U.S. health care was becoming a thicket of vested interests, which, in the event that reform were needed, would prove extremely difficult to trim.

The private voluntary health insurance system of the 1950s was geared toward white men who worked full time in the white collar and industrial sectors. Of the 91 million Americans with some form of medical insurance in 1952, only 7.6 million resided in the southern states from Maryland to Texas.[19] Rural workers of the South and West, many of whom were African

American or itinerant Latino farmworkers, fell largely outside the emerging system of health security. Even where the federal government's role in medical care was largest, such as in congressionally funded community hospitals, Jim Crow laws in southern states continued to repress medical practice liberties for African American physicians and equal access to medical care for black patients.

Commercial insurers and the Blues generally adopted local discriminatory practices. A 1956 Health Insurance Association of America planning document regarded rural inhabitants as "beyond the scope of traditional or even possible or proper concern by private insurers."[20] Women suffered a similar fate because two-thirds of them did not work for wages. And two-thirds of the 23 million women who were gainfully employed worked part time in seasonal jobs or in low-paying service industries where, because of fewer unions and a plentiful labor supply, employers were far less likely to offer health insurance as part of their compensation. Most likely to be covered were women who worked in industry or who were married to an insured man. In the latter case, the woman's coverage hinged on the spousal relationship and the family's ability to pay any additional premiums for dependent coverage. In the event of divorce or insufficient disposable income for supplemental insurance premiums, women and children were usually the first to lose health security.

In addition to its geographic, racial, and gender inequities, voluntary employment-based insurance also discriminated based on class. In 1954 Congress passed and President Eisenhower signed the Internal Revenue Act, which made the long-standing IRS rule on the tax deductibility of group health insurance premiums the law of the land. Now more employers could adopt group plans, confident that any legal challenge to the tax rules would be settled in their favor. As more money flowed to health insurance premiums, the greatest tax breaks went to those with the most valuable coverage and the highest incomes. Workers in the higher income brackets, who therefore would have been subject to higher marginal tax rates on employer/employee-paid insurance premiums, walked away with larger tax breaks than lower-wage workers. In this way, federal tax policy not only played a major role in the growth of employment-based voluntary health insurance, it also contributed to its class inequities.[21]

Both the Americans and the French struggled to expand health care access, but forceful state action was far more likely in France, because *Sécurité Sociale* was a public program and its beneficiaries remained improperly reimbursed for their ambulatory care expenses. The explosive growth of voluntary employment-based health insurance in the United States during the Second World War oriented it away from government programs. Employers, unions, Blue Cross and Blue Shield, and commercial insurers became the appointed slayers of health care costs in the United States. In the absence of national health insurance, Americans brought about what the Committee on the Costs of Medical Care had warned against in 1932. Employment-based voluntary health insurance had bypassed retirees as well as workers and their dependents from poor and unorganized sectors of the economy.[22] In other words, Medicare and Medicaid, far from being a shocking government intrusion into employment-based voluntary health insurance, were, in fact, long-predicted and necessary supplements to it.

France, conversely, had embraced private voluntary health insurance not as a mainstay but as a supplement to its predominant public program, *Sécurité Sociale*. Therein lies the principal divergence between U.S. and French health care after the Second World War. It is within this context that we will examine France's early struggle to contain rising health care costs.

Same Problem, Different Solution

In the late 1950s, retired World War Two generals from the center-right of the political spectrum headed both nations, yet their solutions to the problem of rising health care costs could not have been more different. As troublesome inequities emerged, President Dwight Eisenhower entrusted the ship's bridge to the ingenuity of insurance executives, employers, medical leaders, and union heads. With help from federal hospital construction monies, the deductibility of insurance premiums, and experience rating, they steered the country away from the most damaging premium hikes and toward better medical care for many, but certainly not for all. Yet the U.S. ship lacked a single skipper to survey the distant horizon for potential hazards and to plot a course around them. In 1958 President Charles de Gaulle took the helm of France's ship of state and accepted responsibility for a long-term expansion of health care access and quality, a responsibility that Eisenhower, under the banner of liberty, thought best left in the hands of a diverse, self-interested crew.

To be sure, unlike Eisenhower, de Gaulle assumed power on his own terms, which included a new constitution. He insisted on these changes because of the deep crisis facing the nation. A million French colonists in Algeria, backed by powerful military leaders, threatened to ignore civilian rule and to carry forward a bloody war against Algerian insurgents. France's new constitution created a mixed presidential-parliamentary system that moved power from the legislative to the executive branch. The president now exerted sole power over the conduct of foreign affairs and retained substantial influence over the prime minister, who was drawn from the dominant party in the National Assembly. Adding to de Gaulle's power, his political party scored big victories under the new constitution's first elections, which essentially permitted him to rule by decree during the opening years of his presidency. With the Algerian crisis still very much in play, de Gaulle directed Prime Minister Michel Debré and Minister of Labor Paul Bacon to draft legislation that would bring health care price increases, especially physician fees, under control.

Their May 1960 legislation contained both sticks and carrots for doctors. The stick was unusually large. Under the May law, if negotiations over fee schedules between a departmental *Sécurité Sociale* board and a medical *syndicat* failed, physicians in the department would have two months to decide whether to sign an individual contract with *Sécurité Sociale*. If a physician refused, his patients' reimbursement from *Sécurité Sociale* would be severely restricted, effectively destroying any portion of his practice that relied on *Sécurité Sociale* beneficiaries. The advantages for doctors were smaller but substantial. The May 1960 law continued to allow fee supplements for highly trained and renowned specialists; and to ensure that most departmental negotiations were successful, the government offered a 14 percent rise in health insurance expenditures. This permitted long-overdue hikes in reimbursement rates, especially for general practitioners, and an indexation of medical fees to the general inflation rate. The government also extended some health care and pension benefits to physicians and their dependents.

Prime Minister Michel Debré appealed to doctors "to recognize the modern state, which must act for the improvement of the population's health. . . . Doctors must understand an evolution that is in the nature of things."[23] Yet a substantial portion of the nation's physicians saw nothing natural about the May law's provision for individual contracts. Instead, they viewed it as a wanton attack on their *syndicats,* since any failure in negotiations permitted *Sécurité Sociale* to bypass medical leaders and deal directly with individual practitioners. In response, the CSMF turned to the labor unions, hoping they would see de Gaulle's attack on doctors' *syndicats* as an attack on unions. The medical leader Paul Cibrie lashed out: "I'll ask them [labor leaders] what they would say if they were asked to lead a union of scabs."[24] At first, this appeared to be a promising tactic. France's union chiefs were as mistrustful of de Gaulle's government as U.S. labor leaders were of the Eisenhower administration. But they differed sharply with doctors over whether physicians' *syndicats* were truly unions (like those of industrial workers). This difference revealed diverging ideological views on the question of liberty and equality and thereby on the appropriateness of the government taking action to resolve the problem of rising health care costs.

When Dave Beck, executive vice president of the Teamsters, then affiliated with the AFL, spoke at the AMA's centennial conference, he sounded more like an old friend than a price-conscious consumer, let alone a potential political rival. Beck lambasted Kaiser Health Plans, where patient choice was limited, proclaiming: "I would never, under any circumstances, be a party to an arrangement of any kind whatsoever, which would deny to any man the right to choose the doctor he wishes." Nor did Beck wish to make labor's support for the AMA's professional sovereignty in any way contingent on the continued spread of voluntary insurance. Instead, he dismissed national health insurance as "compulsion and interference with our individual freedom and initiative which lead to State control—dictatorship, Fascism, Communism."

Still, the most telling difference between Beck and his French counterparts came on the question of whether doctors had a union on a par with industrial workers. To Beck, they did. He called the AMA "a union," which, he said, had "every right in the world to protect the interest of [its] members."[25] This could only have left doctors chuckling under their breath, since collective bargaining, which was so sacred to workers' unions, was exactly what doctors were determined to avoid. Their "union" was fighting to protect a physician's individual freedom to set his own fees. Beck confused the Teamsters' collective *economic* power vis-à-vis employers and the AMA's *political* power vis-à-vis the state, which permitted doctors to dictate the modes of production (of health care) and thereby the nature of the market itself.

No French labor leader had any such illusions about the character of the doctors' *syndicats*. When a medical leader wrote to Charles Veillon, head of France's second-largest union, the CGT-FO, in an attempt to enlist his support against de Gaulle's May 1960 law, he found a labor leader who knew what a union was. And it didn't include a professional association like the doctors' Confédération des Syndicats Médicaux Français (CSMF). Veillon responded with a letter of his own in which he poignantly questioned the ideological bases on which physicians opposed the new law. "I believe there's a contradiction between the desire for liberty on the part of practitioners and their surprise, if not indignation, with being given the choice of individual contracts, which their desire for liberty should lead them to find completely acceptable." The "real problem," continued Veillon, "is the antagonism between a system of liberty and a system based on the needs of society." For Veillon, de Gaulle's May law constituted a reasonable compromise between the two, "not because we will follow this government anywhere, but because it has finally joined us on grounds where we have too long remained alone...in a solution that conforms to the general interest."[26] And so it was that, one after another, French labor leaders, including the moderate Christian Democrats, rejected doctors' pleas for "union" solidarity in the face of government action to hold down medical fees.[27]

Physicians received an equally cold shoulder from employers. Throughout the 1940s and 1950s, employers made no secret of their nostalgia for the interwar years, when nonprofit mutual aid societies had served as the country's principal carriers of health insurance.[28] Nevertheless, they came to respect *Sécurité Sociale* when it demonstrated its ability to administer health insurance with lower overhead costs than private nonprofit or commercial insurers. In the face of escalating health care costs, employers instead blamed workers for abusing their access to health care and offered a blanket condemnation of health insurance as "too onerous for the obtained results."[29] They did not blame either hospitals or physicians.

By 1957, however, when the government again floated the idea of binding medical fee schedules, employers were conspicuously neutral, stating that "the Conseil National du Patronat Français will remain outside the debate over the proposed new regulations...of a profession that it does not represent." Employers' neutrality was, in fact, a stinging reversal for doctors, especially since employers also said: "We will attend only to defending our economy against particularly inopportune increases in charges."[30] This was a clear warning to doctors and political leaders that, if they considered raising payroll taxes to pay physicians more, they did so at their peril. Employers had grown weary of haggling over medical fees and inadequate reimbursements from *Sécurité Sociale* to beneficiaries.

Despite their rebuff by workers' unions and employers, doctors in several regions fought the implementation of the May 1960 law with administrative strikes. In reaction to calls for a total walkout, the CSMF's leader, Paul Cibrie, held fast to his pledge that he would sooner resign than authorize a strike targeting patient care. Thus, striking physicians could only refuse to complete the paperwork necessary for the smooth functioning of *Sécurité Sociale*. Although very effective at gumming up the country's health insurance system, the tactic also earned doctors the scorn of patients, whose reimbursements were slowed for lack of proper documentation from doctors' offices. As the date for implementation of the May law neared, increasing numbers of doctors went ahead and signed individual contracts with *Sécurité Sociale*, evoking the wrath of their fellows, who called them "useless shabby scabs, the refuse of the medical profession."[31] Many other physicians, however, believed the government's recourse to individual contracts had been provoked by the intransigence of a few departmental medical leaders. They warned of "defending old, poorly fortified positions" and advocated "indispensable structural reforms" to the practice of medicine, which would safeguard it as a "private *métier*."[32]

The holdouts were concentrated in and around Paris, Lyons, and Orléans. These regions had long exhibited physician resistance to compulsory health insurance, in part because their urban wealth provided more opportunity to create medical practices without patients who relied on *Sécurité Sociale*. Meanwhile, the leadership of the CSMF, knowing it was beat, entered into negotiations with the Gaullist government to improve certain details of the May 1960 law. By November 1960, 85 percent of France's doctors had signed up with *Sécurité Sociale*, either through departmental or individual contracts. This prompted a revolt by hard-liners from the holdout regions, who left the CSMF to create their own professional association, eventually known as the Fédération des Médecins de France (FMF).[33] Indeed, the May 1960 law eventually resulted in the fragmentation of France's medical profession into several associations with sometimes divergent interests, a development that has affected every health care reform since.

After the storm of protest over the May 1960 law had passed, France's health care politics remained turbulent but productive. Despite hard-liners' doomsday predictions, private fee-for-service medical practices remained vibrant and predominant. Physicians' prescriptive freedoms remained unassailable, as did patients' choice of doctor and their direct access to specialists. Moreover, because the May 1960 law pumped additional funds into health care to improve patient reimbursement, doctors witnessed sharp rises in utilization, resulting in even greater fiscal commitments from *Sécurité Sociale*. After its initial jump in 1961 to cover the costs of higher fees associated with the May 1960 law, health insurance spending (in constant francs) rose at an annual rate of just below 12 percent between 1962 and 1967. France's vibrant economy met these rising costs and even permitted legislators to pass something akin to the American Hill-Burton Act of 1946, which opened the way for government investment in hospitals and clinics across the country.[34]

Since the CSMF's most conservative members had left to protest the binding fee schedules and individual contracts, its leaders could now openly endorse a policy of détente with the government. Paul Cibrie retired, and the new CSMF president, Jacques Monier, asserted that "relations between medical practitioners and those responsible for health insurance must be that of an armed peace." But though Monier recognized a state of constant tension, he also rejected the notion that compulsory health insurance was by nature inimical to private practice. "There is no antimony between our free profession and *Sécurité Sociale* . . . for it was the democracies, not the Communist countries, who 'invented' *Sécurité Sociale*."[35] If CSMF membership numbers are any guide, Monier's policy of détente with public authorities satisfied a sizable majority in the profession. Having fallen to a low of 56 percent during the controversy over the May 1960 law, by 1963 CSMF membership had rebounded to 60 percent, while only 17 percent of doctors belonged to rival groups, usually the FMF. Thirteen percent belonged to no association at all.[36] Indeed, Monier felt strong enough to take a hard line in negotiations with *Sécurité Sociale* when fee hikes failed to meet physicians' expectations in 1965.

Doctors' triumph in the 1965 negotiations demonstrated the validity of Monier's "armed peace" approach to professional sovereignty. As long as physicians safeguarded private-practice medicine and acted to assure patient reimbursement under it, they enjoyed broad public support for moderate fee hikes, and thereby held the upper hand with *Sécurité Sociale*.[37] Key to this state of affairs was a continuing expansion of *Sécurité Sociale* to an ever-larger portion of the population. As enrollment grew, beneficiaries could exert tremendous pressure to attain a smoothly functioning health care system, one that included no restrictions on doctors' clinical freedoms or patient choice. In an odd twist of fate, by the late 1960s private-practice medicine in France was bolstered, not hindered, by the continued growth of compulsory public health insurance. In fact, the very success of *Sécurité Sociale* dissolved what had been fierce resistance from groups that had refused to join. With the addition of the agricultural sector in 1961 and of nonfarm self-employed workers in 1966, *Sécurité Sociale* had reached 96 percent of the population by 1970.

Different Problem, Different Solution

Meanwhile, the United States witnessed a twist of its own. By the early 1960s, many employers, hospitals, insurers, and labor and political leaders came to realize that only through government intervention could the vast complex of private voluntary health plans survive. At that time, the United States hit what might be called the 75 percent plateau. Employment-based coverage accounted for 75 percent of all health insurance enrollees. Employers and their employees paid 75 percent of all health insurance premiums. And the Health Insurance Institute estimated that 136 million Americans, or 75 percent of the population, possessed some form of health insurance.[38] Much of the unionized working class, as well as middle- and upper-class professionals—along with their dependents—enjoyed generous health care benefits. The spread of health insurance coverage, however, had slowed to a crawl.

It was increasingly apparent that the aged, unorganized, and poor would never enjoy the same access and benefits without government action. Group health insurance premiums were climbing at 7 percent per year, double the rate of overall inflation between 1950 and 1960; and the price tag for hospital services was rising at four times the general index. Meanwhile, insurers' loss ratios (the ratio of benefits paid out relative to premium income) for nearly all types of group health insurance (the Blues, Kaiser, and the commercials) now topped 90 percent. Gone were the days (the immediate postwar years) when insurance companies could count on retaining as much as 25 percent of their premium revenue, part of which was kept as profit, the rest returned to employers (sometimes workers) in the form of dividends. With insurers squeezed and labor leaders and employers alike clamoring to hold down health care costs, the poor and elderly found themselves in an impossible position. Even Eisenhower and the AMA recognized the danger.

In 1960 they both supported a congressional proposal by Senator Robert Kerr of Oklahoma and Representative Wilbur Mills of Arkansas. The Kerr-Mills bill offered means-tested health coverage in collaboration with state governments, a program that would eventually become known as "Medicaid." The elderly, however, required an altogether different solution. In retirement, they lacked the all-important connection to employment on which the U.S. system of health security had been built. Further, according to insurance underwriters, the elderly had high medical care utilization rates and thus represented a much higher risk. Their participation drove up the price of experience-rated policies, which were increasingly preferred by employers and labor unions to combat premium rises.

Exactly for this reason, labor leaders and employers parted ways with the AMA and supported President John F. Kennedy's compulsory health insurance initiative for Social Security beneficiaries. Still, Republican opponents of Kennedy's proposal wanted to know what was wrong with collectively bargained voluntary health insurance for retirees. Why, they wanted to know, had labor unions "abandoned Samuel Gompers [the AFL founder] who opposed compulsion in fields such as this." In testimony before the House Ways and Means Committee, AFL-CIO president George Meany responded to this question by effectively throwing his lot in with employers: "Very few industries are able to stand the financial costs.... [We have] been unable to solve this particular problem through collective bargaining."[39]

What employers in France and the United States feared most was a health care breakdown that would result in wholesale reform, leading to what they both called "socialized medicine."[40] Employers in both nations preferred employment-based health insurance and private-practice medicine as long as it was not too expensive. But if health care became separated from employment, as in, say, a British-style national health service, U.S. employers stood to lose a useful lever to retain skilled workers and to promote employee loyalty. Likewise, French employers enjoyed allotted seats on *Sécurité Sociale* boards, seats whose justification would surely erode if payrolls no longer served as the source of health insurance premiums. Thus, in both nations, employers consistently assessed the effect of government intervention based on whether it would stabilize the system and safeguard their influence. Or would the proposed government action provide a slippery slope toward more state control of health care? Just as French employers refused to side with doctors when de Gaulle moved to enforce medical fee schedules in May 1960, so most U.S. employers opposed the AMA in 1965 on Medicare.[41] U.S. employers judged that a strong but limited dose of government compulsion could safeguard the predominantly private and voluntary nature of U.S. health care.

Many U.S. and French physicians also employed remarkably similar rhetoric in the 1960s in their attempts to block government action. AMA leaders warned of "socialized medicine for every man, woman, and child," while the CSMF railed against "a government takeover of medicine." French medical leaders claimed that the binding fee schedules instituted by de Gaulle would ruin "the humanitarian traditions that we have always respected." U.S. medical leaders likewise predicted Medicare "would destroy the concepts of individual and family responsibility." And, as in previous health care reform debates, French and U.S. physicians characterized the proposed reforms as utterly foreign and sure to bring disaster.[42]

A Parisian medical leader had claimed that, if de Gaulle's fee schedules were approved, France would be following "the example of Russia, England,

and Germany" and that "patients would soon find that medical offices were open only 9 to 12 and 2 to 5, and were staffed by health officers.... No house calls, no urgent care assured." An AMA board member confidently asserted that his visit to England to "see how socialized medicine works," had "confirm[ed] [his] suspicions that the British system becomes more and more distasteful to the people—the patients and the physicians" every day. AMA president Leonard Larson similarly warned that Medicare would be the first step toward "socialized medicine...a disruption of the doctor-patient relationship, delays in admissions to hospitals; waiting lists for various operations and therapies; regimentation of medical practice;... availability of medical facilities and personnel—in other words, medicine in action on a government run, assembly line basis."[43]

What was overlooked in all this hyperbole was that the best example for each nation to study would have been the other. To better understand how compulsory insurance might influence the values and function of private fee-for-service medicine, AMA leaders could have done no better than to examine France. Likewise, if CSMF leaders had truly wanted to understand the effect of unregulated medical fees on patients and coverage, they would have done well to look at U.S. health care. Yet U.S. and French medical leaders were looking abroad not for instructive experiences but for rhetorical ammunition to fight political battles. What doctors really hoped to sell politicians and the public was the idea that the proposed reform was, as the historian Colin Gordon puts it, "the toe in the door" to ever more government intrusion.[44] But neither the public nor the politicians were buying. In France, de Gaulle succeeded in forcing doctors to retreat on the issue of medical fees. In the United States, President Johnson's reelection in 1964 delivered a Democratic landslide to Congress that fundamentally changed the outlook for opponents of compulsory insurance for the elderly.

In launching his Medicare initiative in 1961, John Kennedy had stood up to the AMA, but he remained fearful of it. By contrast, his successor, Lyndon Johnson, exhibited nothing but disdain for the political might of doctors. In this he resembled de Gaulle, who during his hiatus from politics in the 1950s could only observe the arrogance with which physicians manipulated *Sécurité Sociale*. Once returned to power, and having announced his initiative to rein in doctors' fees, de Gaulle answered with arrogance of his own and remarked to physicians: "I saved France on a colonel's pay. For the billions I pay you, surely you can give me better health care!" Johnson, conversely, had grown up in central Texas and preferred farm analogies. On the eve of the Medicare battle, he confided to AFL-CIO leader Georges

Meany: "Have you ever fed chickens[?]...Chickens are real dumb. They eat and eat and eat and they never stop. Why they start shitting at the same time they're eating, and before you know it, they're knee deep in their own shit. Well, the AMA's the same. They've been eating and eating nonstop and now they're knee deep in their own shit and everybody knows it."[45] In taking on the AMA, Johnson not only relied on a greater Democratic majority in Congress, he also correctly calculated that physicians would find little support from other health care interests.

When the AMA turned to hospitals in search of support in their battle against Medicare legislation, they found only ambivalence. The American Hospital Association was a case in point. Many of its members believed, like the AMA, that Medicare represented an unwarranted government program that would become a springboard for more damaging intervention down the road. As the battle unfolded, however, an increasing number of hospitals became "ready to accept the Social Security principle because they could see no other way to get the needed money" to care for the aged. Equally problematic for medical leaders was that the hospitals' advocacy of Medicare included an insistence that specialists whose practices lay wholly within the confines of hospitals—for example, pathologists, radiologists, and anesthesiologists—be included in the hospital portion of the bill. This position evoked a sharp response from AMA president Donovan Ward, who remarked that "medical care is the responsibility of physicians, not hospitals....If [they] are included...they will be subject to curbing and direction by government employees, untrained in medicine seeking to meet their primary responsibility toward the budget in the only way open to them, through control of services."[46] The conflict between medical leaders and hospital administrators over how to bill for "in-house" doctors recalled the struggles between the early hospital service plans and the AMA in the 1930s. As at that time, the weight of Blue Cross eventually proved decisive in deciding the issue in favor of hospitals. In fact, the proposed role of the Blues and commercial insurers in the whole of the Medicare program significantly influenced the legislative battle and its outcome.

Early on, health insurers stood alongside the AMA in opposition to Medicare, accusing the Kennedy administration of underestimating—correctly, as it turns out—the full price tag of the program. Ideologically, they assumed that "any type of federal program...would include intolerable influence and regulation by the federal government [and]...the likelihood of future expansion of the federal program to younger ages or to other areas of benefits."[47] But like the AHA, the Health Insurance Association of

America (HIAA) was an umbrella organization whose members hailed from diverse sectors of the insurance industry. Over the course of the debate, many large Blue Cross plans became convinced that Medicare legislation would enable them to defend themselves against the growing incursion of commercial insurers into their business and, in so doing, help them preserve community-rated hospital insurance.[48]

Meanwhile, commercial insurers, probably more than anyone, understood the technical reasons why many elderly and poor citizens would remain uninsurable without government action beyond the Kerr-Mills legislation approved in 1960. Like employers, they came to understand that government programs that took care of the elderly (Medicare) and the poor (Medicaid) actually reinforced private employment-based voluntary insurance for nearly everyone else. And once it became clear that Medicare would employ private insurers to help administer the new program, the health insurers' position quickly switched from ambivalence to active participation in shaping the legislation. The role of intermediary between patient, provider, and the federal government was a vein of gold that health insurers showed themselves especially adept at exploiting. With no underwriting risk to worry about, the Blues and commercial insurers both sought to capture lucrative administrative contracts for as many plans, patients, and hospitals as possible.

Despite being abandoned by some of their erstwhile allies, the AMA mounted an attack against the Medicare bill reminiscent of Napoleon's last battle at Waterloo—grand and impressive but still not enough. In an attempt to overcome negative public opinion and the political forces arrayed against them, medical leaders bought quarter-page ads in seven thousand dailies, full-page ads in every major metropolitan newspaper and most major weeklies, thirty national one-minute television spots, and hundreds more in local TV markets. When all was said and done, the AMA had spent 2 million dollars, more than the next nine largest national political lobbies combined.[49] But all the AMA's firepower could not overcome the attitudes of employers, hospitals, and insurers, each of whom foresaw a different advantage for themselves in government intervention.

Democrats had gained thirty-two new House seats in the 1964 congressional elections, permitting them to expand their majority on the all-important Ways and Means Committee, whose approval was vital if the bill was to pass. Since the late years of Franklin Roosevelt's presidency, Republicans and conservative Southern Democrats had been able to block Democrats' social reform bills; but the political winds had now shifted strongly in favor of reformers. Ways and Means Committee chair Wilbur Mills of Arkansas adroitly switched from opponent to advocate of Medicare in order to manage (and therefore influence) the bill.

Perhaps because he was so familiar with opponents' arguments, Mills played his role brilliantly. He cleverly suggested that a single bill should contain all three of the alternatives then before the committee, creating what Health, Education, and Welfare (HEW) secretary Wilbur Cohen called "a three layer cake." Medicare Part A would provide hospital insurance funded by an increase in the Social Security wage levy. Part B would offer voluntary insurance for physician services, to be paid for by beneficiary premiums and the federal treasury. The cake's bottom layer, which became Medicaid, was a more generous version of the Kerr-Mills law of 1960 that supplied medical care to the poor.[50] Mills's bill survived essentially intact to become the revised version approved by the House (307 to 116) and the Senate (70 to 24) on 27 July 1965. In a tribute to President Harry Truman's unsuccessful efforts to enact national health insurance, Johnson signed the Medicare bill into law in Independence, Missouri, three days later.[51] France and the United States both experienced forceful government-led reforms during the 1960s. When the dust had cleared, two fundamental similarities between their health care systems remained and two divergent trends had been reinforced, both with important implications for later reforms.

Fee-for-service private-practice medicine survived the government interventions to emerge as hallowed as ever in both nations. To be sure, the French law of May 1960 subjected French physicians to explicit and more constraining fee schedules. Yet they continued to bill their patients directly and they remained free from utilization reviews of their diagnoses, treatment, and prescriptions. Thus, in practice, French doctors substantially retained control of their incomes because of their still-unquestioned ability to *intensify* their practice of medicine, that is, to conduct more tests and procedures, for which they could be assured payment. Meanwhile, their patients' choice of doctor and direct access to specialists also remained fully protected, as did doctor-patient confidentiality.

Back in the United States, despite AMA leaders' dire predictions of what would happen if Medicare were enacted, U.S. doctors gained generous federal guarantees of private-practice medicine. Far from pushing their legislative victory into a broader offensive to control health care costs, U.S. government officials embraced the liberties of fee-for-service practice. Even when Blue Cross president Walter McNerney suggested that negotiated fee schedules, which by then were functioning smoothly in France, would be the best way to comply with Medicare's directive to deliver uniform benefits at a "reasonable" cost, HEW officials demurred, saying they would "get us into the touchy doctor area."[52]

Instead, Medicare adopted prevailing billing practices, notably "usual, customary, and reasonable" fees whose inflationary effects were well known. Likewise, hospital services under Medicare were billed on a "cost plus" basis; hospitals simply billed for their services and tacked on an extra percentage for depreciation of plant and equipment.[53] Thus, while both nations safeguarded private medicine, they did so in blunt and inefficient ways. During the first year of Medicare's implementation, hospital charges rose 16.5 percent and physician fees were up 7.8 percent—double the increases of previous years. France had certainly made greater progress in restraining medical fee inflation, but both countries would soon have to revisit how health insurers dealt with physicians and hospitals.

Reforms did not substantially alter the central role of employment in health security in either nation. Because *Sécurité Sociale* was rapidly being extended to an ever-greater proportion of the French population, including those with irregular employment, the negative effects of employment-based insurance were not as keenly felt as in the United States. Nevertheless, many French beneficiaries remained reliant on their employers to purchase supplemental mutual society health coverage that made up the difference between *Sécurité Sociale* reimbursements and physician fees. Also, the continued reliance on payroll levies that took a flat percentage of workers' wages without regard for their overall income reinforced the inequity of health care financing. U.S. Medicare had the same effect on health care financing because, like Social Security contributions, the Medicare wage levy was a regressive tax, taking a larger bite of disposable income from low-wage workers than from their better-paid coworkers.

The difference between Medicare and Medicaid perpetuated the distinction between "deserving" and "less deserving" citizens to a much greater extent than existed in France's employment-based health insurance. Although current employment was not required for Medicare beneficiaries, eligibility depended on having amassed ten years of Social Security contributions. Nor did mere eligibility suffice. Medicare beneficiaries had to pay premiums to obtain coverage for physician fees (Part B), and even then patients remained responsible for some portion of their medical bills, including 100 percent of prescription drugs. The ineligible and those without sufficient funds to make use of Medicare Part B turned to Medicaid, whose means testing and lower physician payments added up to less patient choice, under a stigmatized poverty assistance program for the "less deserving."

Moreover, in the South, where distinctions had long been made along racial lines, hundreds of local hospitals viewed their African American Medicare and Medicaid patients as the least deserving of all. Although hospitals fell under the jurisdiction of the Civil Rights Act of 1964, which outlawed discrimination in programs that received federal funds, enforcement by federal officials was haphazard at best. Blind to the historic events unfolding before them, HEW administrators placed their agency's parochial interests above an ultimately more important movement for civil rights. They wanted, above all, a smooth launch to Medicare, which they undeniably achieved. Nine out of ten eligible Social Security beneficiaries signed up for the supplemental medical insurance available to them under Medicare Part B, and one in five elderly Americans entering the hospital in 1966 did so under the program. But in the South, black patients continued to face separate entrances and waiting rooms, and unequal hospital services. A 1971 federal government report lamented that discrimination by providers of Medicare-funded services in the South was so rampant that it made "a mockery of the efforts of many men and women who have fought for civil rights."[54] Medicare and Medicaid's shortcomings notwithstanding, the 1965 legislation represented a remarkable achievement in extending wider access to health care in the United States.

Yet Medicare and Medicaid also represent the antithesis of France's health care reforms of 1945 and 1960. The French reforms were milestones in the progressive expansion of health security to the entire population, which had begun with industrial workers in 1930. Despite the hopes of some officials within the Johnson administration, public health insurance for the elderly and a means-tested program for the poor proved a poor springboard for further reform. In fact, Medicare and Medicaid were purposely crafted to discourage future federal health insurance initiatives. Wilbur Mills, who received a standing ovation on the House floor for his leadership in passing the Medicare legislation, explained that his inclusion of voluntary insurance for physician services (Part B) "would build a fence around the Medicare program." Those who wished to extend Medicare Part B to other sectors of the population could not simply draw on Social Security funds to do so. Instead, they would have to provide a separate funding source, to essentially create a whole new program, a very high hurdle to jump indeed in U.S. health care politics.[55]

Reflections on the Choice of Public or Private

By 1970, medicine's twentieth-century achievements would have been as astounding to a physician of 1900 as the 1969 moon landing would have been to the Wright brothers. Meningitis, tuberculosis, polio, smallpox, and most general infections had been substantially conquered. Surgeons opened hearts to clear passages and exposed the brain to remove tumors. By having their blood replaced, newborn babies who would have died in 1900 could now be saved. An array of waves and rays probed organs, tissues, and cells. Psychiatrists prescribed pharmaceuticals, correcting mental illnesses previously regarded as incurable.[56] Yet the question of who enjoyed access to these stupendous medical breakthroughs and who paid for them remained far from settled, as national leaders grappled with competing priorities and approaches to health care.

For all their good intentions, postwar U.S. labor leaders bought a fake whose imperfections became tragically clear within a few decades. Despite the example of French (and most other western European) labor leaders, who insisted on legislation that would guarantee workers' health security, most U.S. unions gave their campaigns for national health insurance second billing. Their headline act was the securing of generous private health and welfare benefits at the collective bargaining table, by winning experience-rated insurance. As successful as this strategy was in the 1950s and 1960s, by the 1980s it had proved a sham. As U.S. job growth moved from the manufacturing to the service sectors, the health insurance that union and nonunion members alike had come to take for granted now became vulnerable. A study conducted between 1985 and 1991 showed that, for every one hundred *manufacturing* jobs lost, two hundred and twenty-four workers and dependents lost their health insurance. For every one hundred new *service* jobs, only forty workers and their dependents gained coverage.[57] Little wonder that by the 1990s health security had become a permanent anxiety across much of the U.S. labor force.

Although French workers could feel far more secure about their access to good health care, the law of May 1960 failed to control health care costs as anticipated. In fact, just as CSMF leader Monier had claimed, the law created a harsh new reality of constant conflict between physicians and the government. In a major restructuring of *Sécurité Sociale* in 1967, labor leaders, employers, and government officials raised the health insurance wage levy from 6 to 6.5 percent, the first hike since 1945. Yet what hurt more was the simultaneous decrease in reimbursement for many ambulatory care procedures, from 80 to 70 percent. Inpatient hospital expenses continued to be covered at 100 percent. Legislators also recast *Sécurité Sociale* governing boards to give employers the same number of seats as union leaders. Despite the outrage of union leaders at the time, it soon became apparent to employers and labor leaders alike that, as in the United States, the principal challenge to achieving health security was not their opponent but rather the rising cost of medical care.

In a 1944 report, the founding father of *Sécurité Sociale*, Pierre Laroque, had calmly projected steady rises in health care expenditures that would keep pace with a growing economy and extended coverage but would not outrun them. As he had predicted, health insurance coverage more than doubled, from 45 to 95 percent of the population by 1967, but health care spending grew at twice the rate on average as that at which *Sécurité Sociale* was extended to new beneficiaries, far outpacing general economic growth.[58] As a result, health care has consumed a larger and larger portion of France's national income every year since 1947. Similarly daunting statistics have also weighed on the U.S. economy. Even as their approaches diverged, attempts to control spending moved to the fore in both countries after 1970.

7

COST CONTROL MOVES TO THE FORE, 1970–2000

Even if good health has no price, we cannot deny that it has a cost.

Minister of Health Jacques Barrot, *Le Concours Médical*, 1 November 1980

The late 1960s and 1970s were a time of profound social upheaval in France and the United States. The war in Vietnam waged by the United States provoked widespread protests there and in Europe, especially in France where, it should be remembered, French troops had already shed their own and Vietnamese blood before withdrawing in 1954. Although French student protesters identified with their U.S. counterparts about the war, they were also focused on the inadequacy of schools to meet the demands of the bulging baby boom generation. Add to these developments a critical new awareness of environmental destruction and the Watergate scandal and the combined result was a popular outpouring of discontent that indicted the French and U.S. political classes as well as "the system" to which they paid respect.

The oil price shocks delivered by the Organization of the Petroleum Exporting Countries (OPEC) in the 1970s heightened the public's sense of crisis. As gasoline prices skyrocketed, it was plain to everyone that a vital commodity for life in industrialized nations was in short supply. The resulting worldwide economic slowdown was especially hard-felt in France. Indeed, for French economic historians, 1975 marked the end of *les trente glorieuses*—a glorious thirty-year stretch of economic growth. As stagflation and recession fell over Europe and the United States, leaders on both sides of the Atlantic sought solutions: conservation, lower speed limits, higher gasoline taxes to promote public transit, and a renewed search for energy sources. A new generation of American and French people, who had not experienced the meager days of the Depression or the Second World War, became painfully aware of their costly way of life.

These developments provide a critical setting for our story about health care in France and the United States after 1970. Until this time, and despite their differences, virtually all U.S. and French health care reformers viewed the extension and improvement of insurance coverage, whether publicly or privately financed, as their single most important goal. In the United States, the creation of Medicare and Medicaid in 1965 was hailed as a great success, with scant attention paid to health care's obvious inflationary tendencies. In France, the extension of *Sécurité Sociale* benefits to the self-employed and agricultural sectors in the 1960s marked a vast expansion of the welfare state. In both nations, political leaders, labor unions, and even insurers and some employers advocated more generous medical service entitlements with little regard for controlling costs.

By the early 1970s, however, when both countries were suffering from recession and the quickening pace of health care inflation, efficiency and cost control had moved to the fore.[1] Waste was out. Conservation was in. But conserving medical care resources through the improvement of physicians' productivity, limitations on patient access, and the assessment of health care outcomes is not a purely technical challenge. As governments, insurers, and employers sought closer management of previously unmanaged medical decision making, they laid bare historical tensions between powerful health care interests. Further, by their very nature, constraints on health care utilization threatened patient choice and physicians' clinical freedoms, which were social and cultural ideals to which both nations aspired. Proposals to enforce water or energy conservation sometimes provoke political battles. Health care rationing always does.

Prices without a Market

In 1969, President Richard Nixon warned of "a crippling inflation in medical costs causing vast increases in government health expenditures for little return... [and rising] private health insurance premiums." Between 1968 and 1970, Medicare enrollment had risen 19 percent while spending outlays had jumped 57 percent.[2] A leading official at France's *Sécurité Sociale*, Clément Michel, added an explanation to Nixon's expression of alarm: "There's no financial problem with health insurance but rather an economic problem in health care, born of the extraordinary progress of medicine."[3]

Health care inflation appeared to be built-in and enduring in both countries. Between 1960 and 1993, consumer price inflation in the United States rose at an annual average rate of 4.9 percent, but health care costs rose more than twice as fast, at an annual average rate of just over 11 percent. France suffered a similar disparity between the general inflation rate and medical price hikes. There annual health care increases averaged 15 percent between 1960 and 1978, while the general inflation rate averaged only 6.3 percent. Already in 1970, France and the United States had two of the most expensive health care systems in the world, spending 5.6 and 7.4 percent respectively of their GDP. By 1987, France's proportion devoted to health care had risen to 8.6 percent, outstripping every other major western European country. But if the French appeared profligate among their fellow Europeans, the United States had moved into a class of extravagance all its own, expending 11.2 percent of national income on health care in 1987.

Both countries had gone on a hospital construction spree after the Second World War. The Hill-Burton Act of 1946 had allocated billions of dollars from general tax revenues to build community hospitals across the country. U.S. hospital care accounted for 53 percent of the nation's health care spending by 1974. France was not far behind. A hike in *Sécurité Sociale* payroll taxes in 1945 and 1967, along with allocations from the health ministry, provided ample funds for similar projects. Once built, the new facilities in both nations were more expensive to operate than older hospitals, since they had far more private and semiprivate rooms, as opposed to open wards. Overall, hospital spending (construction and operations) accounted for the lion's share of the health care spending increases during the immediate postwar decades. By 1977, fully half of all French health care outlays were devoted to the hospital sector, up from 39 percent in 1950.[4]

Fresh breakthroughs in medical science, technology, and pharmaceuticals also drove health care inflation. This progress, in turn, affected both the practice of medicine and patients' attitudes toward malady and health. With fantastic new tools, techniques, and therapies at their disposal, doctors could hardly be blamed for becoming more aggressive clinicians. If something could be done, they did it. If a second test would eliminate a small uncertainty, they ordered it, even if it was just as costly as the first. Second and even third medical opinions became far more common, despite their high cost. In France, a term was coined, *le nomadisme médical*, to describe patients who sought diagnoses and prescriptions from a second, third, and even fourth specialist for the same condition, all of which were covered by *Sécurité Sociale* without question. Meanwhile, new machines—linear accelerators, echocardiographs, lasers, and diagnostic imaging devices (such as Computed Tomography (CT) and Magnetic Resonance Imaging (MRI)—required new subspecialists to operate them.[5] The new specialties, however, were just part of a much larger explosion in scientific discovery that transformed medical knowledge and its application.[6]

During the last third of the twentieth century, biological and medical research became multibillion-dollar international endeavors, whose latest results were quickly shared across the globe. By 1998, the online medical library, *Medline*, received twenty thousand new articles per month, drawn from three thousand refereed journals worldwide.[7] The explosion of knowledge, accompanied by advances in information technology, made possible the treatment of poorly understood pathologies and many more that had previously been considered untreatable. For example, hospital intensive care units, armed with improved ventilators, more sensitive monitoring devices, and the latest life-sustaining drugs administered intravenously became so successful at keeping patients alive that admitting physicians were unable to keep up with their care. Hence, more and more hospitals have turned to a new subspecialist, the intensivist, a specially trained medical doctor, to oversee patient care in the intensive care unit (ICU). These innovations benefit the sick and injured; moreover, as a result of the accelerating advances in curative medicine, the public has come to believe that little is beyond the capabilities of the medical complexes that dot their cities and countryside.

By 1980, with fifteen thousand operations a year, the near-miraculous procedure of open-heart surgery had become almost mundane in France. For a short time, the public marveled at this stupendous advance in cardiology, but the price of it all escaped them. In 1980, open-heart surgery cost more than seven times the maximum annual *Sécurité Sociale* contribution, an amazing statistic if one remembers that only sixty years earlier, medical bills were deemed a practically inconsequential burden of illness. Early health insurance initiatives had been far more concerned with protecting the ill from the risk of lost wages; but by 1970 the medical revolution had turned the world on its head. The new order called for increasingly invasive, complex, and expensive procedures. In the United States, the number of surgeons nearly doubled, from 58,000 in 1970 to 106,000 in 1985, far exceeding the population growth rate of the United States.[8] Yet the price of surgery continued to rise far more quickly than the general inflation rate. How could that be? Should not the greatly increased supply of surgeons have meant lower prices for surgery, or at least a slowing in their rate of increase?

In fact, with just such thinking in mind, political leaders on both sides of the Atlantic, responding to the quickening pace of health care inflation after 1970, stressed various proposals that sought to "take advantage of market forces." Yet, in contrast to the 1920s, when the arrival of more physicians or the building of additional medical facilities in a particular locale sometimes pushed medical fees downward, the post–Second World War era has demonstrated that health care has little in common with what most people define as a market.

Put simply, a market is a self-regulating mechanism for the allocation of resources, where sellers compete to provide the best price or the highest quality, and buyers have sufficient knowledge to make rational decisions in their own best interest. To begin with, the supply of health care is largely in the hands of professions whose licensing and training requirements create effective monopolies in the provision of care. Meanwhile, on the demand side, patients rarely possess sufficient expertise or experience to make rational decisions in their best interest; and even if they possess such knowledge, many are so seriously impaired by their medical condition that they cannot make use of it. Instead, in direct violation of market sense, patients rely on the seller to tell them why and what to buy, that is, their diagnosis and their treatment. Then, when it comes time to pay, a third party (the insurer), who has been outside the seller-buyer (doctor-patient) relationship, pays the bill. Last, while the real price of most other products, such as automobiles or computers, declined substantially as improvements in technology and production techniques became available, health care has tended to increase in cost.[9]

In 1970, the French public health expert Georges Malignac conducted an economic analysis of U.S. health care for France's leading medical journal, *Le Concours Médical*. He concluded that "the problem is not only to figure out how to halt the rising price of care, but how to reorganize the existing medical and paramedical institutions in order to make them more efficient; however, that would directly challenge the reigning dogma." By "reigning dogma" he meant the broad practice and billing liberties enjoyed by private-practice physicians and the generous cost-plus reimbursements received by hospitals. Malignac did not attempt to hide the fact that such problems also pertained to France: "One cannot help being struck by certain similarities between economic studies of medicine and the cost of health care on both sides of the Atlantic." That led directly to a conclusion addressed to the French medical profession. "It appears to me that the country of free enterprise [the United States] is in dire need of some [health care] planning. Those in our country who wish a return to the good old days of our grandfathers should take note."[10]

Malignac encapsulated the dilemma facing both countries: you can't solve health care price inflation without changing the way patients and practitioners use medical resources. Yet in both countries all attempts to reform health care utilization inevitably sparked debate over patient choice, medical practice liberties, and the quality and equality of care.

Health Care Planning for Cost Control Efforts in France

Even though France was and remains home to fiercely independent private practitioners, the country has long embraced a modicum of state-directed planning of its economy. After the Second World War, successive governments adroitly guided economic growth using a series of plans.[11] Their control levers over the economy were large nationalized firms, the gas, electricity, coal, and banking industries, and financial services. Dubbed "indicative plans" by one political scientist to distinguish them from the authoritarian documents once produced by the Soviet Union, French plans were the state's way of pressuring commercial and industrial leaders to line up behind the government's economic growth strategy.[12]

French planning also included contingencies to avoid social conflict, especially crippling strikes that could hamper growth. As *Sécurité Sociale* played an increasingly important role in preserving social peace, and as health care's share of the overall economy grew, it was only a matter of time before medicine itself became a subject of interest at the Ministry of Planning. In 1970, government planners invited medical leaders to participate in deliberations over the country's sixth plan since the end of the war. They hoped to facilitate the negotiation of a national *convention* between physicians and *Sécurité Sociale*, thereby replacing the numerous departmental agreements that had been negotiated since the creation of compulsory health insurance in 1930. A uniform fee schedule, insisted planners, could serve to make the country's jumble of medical care compensation arrangements fairer.

In principle, most doctors agreed. In fact, leaders of France's largest doctors' association, the Confédération des Syndicats Médicaux Français

(CSMF), who in 1960 had ultimately compromised with government officials on binding fees, viewed a national *convention* as a way to call to account many of the Paris and Lyons physicians who had split the medical profession. In 1960, these doctors had denounced the CSMF, claiming it had sold out the freedoms of private-practice medicine; in response, they had created their own group, which came to be called the Fédération des Médecins de France (FMF). Over the course of the subsequent decade, however, many of these same doctors signed individual contracts with *Sécurité Sociale* to pursue part-time private practices while relying on salaried hospital positions for most of their income. CSMF leaders viewed this as hypocritical, especially from those who espoused such disruptively purist positions on private-practice medicine. They saw a national *convention* as a way to diminish the role of individual physician contracts with *Sécurité Sociale* and to reunify the profession under their own leadership.[13]

Government planners also found support among employers for a national *convention*. By 1970 French employers were finally ready to openly question the appropriateness of physicians' near-absolute clinical freedoms under a system of public health insurance that now appeared destined to reach the entire population. Doctors' status as small businesspeople had previously restrained the larger business community from calling for more government regulation of private-practice medicine. Prior to the mid-1960s, the nation's leading employer associations had limited themselves to making clear their opposition to increased payroll taxes. Now, in the face of persistent medical inflation, employers abandoned their reticence; they openly attacked doctors' monopoly over medical decision making. As one official put it, "an employer offensive... had begun.... Physicians had no choice: either they were going to let others regulate their practices or they could participate in the promulgation of those regulations [through the national *convention*]."[14]

A leaked government memo even advocated replacing fee-for-service billing with capitated and salaried compensation. Forced to explain the memo to a scandalized medical press, the secretary of the health planning committee, Michel Flamme, struck back. He insisted that his memo only said aloud what had been whispered in private for a long time, namely, that fee-for-service remuneration encourages unneeded procedures and hinders "the practice of quality medicine: the more time a practitioner spends with his patients, the better his diagnosis, the more judicious his prescriptions, but the smaller his pay." Why not, reasoned Flamme, consider all types of payment methods that might improve preventive and curative care?

With their traditional billing practices under threat, doctors were forced to concede what had hitherto been anathema: the individualized monitoring of medical decision making by *Sécurité Sociale*. If judged consistently, egregiously, and indefensibly wasteful by a panel of peers, a doctor could be excluded from participation in *Sécurité Sociale*. That is, his or her patients would no longer be eligible for reimbursement of medical fees, a sanction that would effectively ruin the practice of all but the most renowned doctors.[15]

In return for this concession to cost control, or what medical leaders preferred to call "self-discipline," physicians gained a long-sought protection for fee-for-service medicine. The government forbade the creation of primary care clinics by regional *Sécurité Sociale* authorities. Medical leaders had fought a running battle with mutual society–run clinics, where doctors had been employed on a salaried and capitated basis since the 1930s. Because in many ways regional *Sécurité Sociale* boards constituted the successors to interwar mutual societies, the prohibition marked a substantial victory for autonomous private practitioners.[16]

Even more striking, the circumstances under which doctors could exceed standard fees were extended. Previously, departmental agreements usually included language that permitted a physician to adjust his fees "according to the wealth of the patient." But for practical reasons, physicians rarely invoked this right. The new fee waiver depended not on the patient's financial status but on the nature of the medical circumstances at hand and the experience and qualifications of the attending physician. For example, a physician with special training or extensive experience in the treatment of critical lung conditions could charge a patient with acute respiratory edema substantially more than the standard fee. What is more, a condition could be deemed to be of medical complexity simply if it called for "psycho-social approaches requiring an extended interview of the patient."[17] The additional fees, however, were borne by the patient (or her supplementary insurer) and not by *Sécurité Sociale*. Instead of striking directly at health care inflation, the new fee waivers simply shifted the burden of who pays. The hope was that this would curtail demand and thereby dampen prices. By the end of 1970, 89 percent of French doctors had agreed to the national *convention*; 96 percent had done so by the end of 1974.[18] The vast majority of doctors were apparently willing to countenance the surveillance of their medical decision making if by agreeing they gained something in return. We will see a comparable quid pro quo played out on a far vaster scale in the United States, with the rise of managed care in the 1990s.

The existence of a dominant public insurer, *Sécurité Sociale*, had motivated France's earlier actions to slow government spending on health care. Yet the French state's enhanced role did not necessarily translate into effective measures against the broader problem of health care inflation. The contradictory impulses we have witnessed since the beginning of our story—between liberties of patient choice and medical practice on the one hand and equality of access on the other—continued to divide the public and hamper reform. Hovering over it all was the question of whether France should expand the role of government by creating a British-style national health service, thereby doing away with its reliance on fee-for-service private practitioners altogether. The *Sécurité Sociale* governing board approved the new national *convention*, but its twelve-to-five split vote foreshadowed tensions over health care ideals that would remain unresolved through the end of the century.

France's largest union, the CGT, opposed the national *convention* because of the greatly expanded prerogatives it granted physicians to exceed standard fee schedules. Its *Sécurité Sociale* representative explained: "We often find ourselves on the same side as doctors, defending their social protections, the adjustment of their fees for inflation, and a fair tax treatment of their earnings. [Yet we] cannot accept the new changes…particularly the right of a physician to exceed fee schedules when he alone considers himself to have acquired greater medical knowledge."[19]

In favor of the new *convention*, large employers and agricultural interests took a carrot-and-stick approach to health care cost control. They readily endorsed the ideals of private-practice medicine, especially the entrepreneurialism of autonomous practitioners, with whom they claimed an ideological affinity. Yet, completely out of character with their usual laissez-faire views, some employers also insisted that a British-style, government-run national health service remained a viable option. For the time being, however, the monitoring of physicians' treatment practices should serve "to alert doctors to economic conditions that cannot be ignored." Or, in the words of the agricultural representative, "We take very seriously our responsibility to examine the creation of a truly national health service.…The future of private-practice medicine is in the hands not of social or political institutions but in those of doctors themselves."[20]

Employers' warning to physicians that they might support the creation of a national health service was founded on the growing disparity between French and British health care expenditures. Great Britain had launched its National Health Service at virtually the same moment as France had created *Sécurité Sociale* after the Second World War. And despite Britain's more rapid progress toward achieving universal coverage, it was not experiencing the same levels of health care inflation. Britain's health care spending grew from 3.9 percent of GDP in 1960 to just 6 percent in 1985, while France increased its share of GDP devoted to health care from 4.2 to 8.4 percent during the same years.

Yet the picture was more complex. This was not just a conflict between employers who wished to trim health care costs and beneficiaries who insisted on continued equality of access and fees. If some employers were willing to threaten doctors with the prospect of a national health service, others remained staunchly opposed to a health service, and not only because it represented "socialized medicine." It would have also meant upending the "social partners" construction of *Sécurité Sociale*, which granted employers significant administrative power, and replacing it with direct state control. Joining these employers was France's second-largest union, the Force Ouvrière (FO), which represented many health care workers. Its representative on the *Sécurité Sociale* board supported the new *convention* with rhetoric that could have been lifted straight from a medical leader's speech from the 1930s. He explicitly embraced the nation's tradition of "private-practice medicine characterized by free choice, liberty of prescription, fee for service, and respect of medical confidentiality."[21] Meanwhile, the French Communist Party blasted the 1971 *convention* on the grounds that the monitoring of physician treatment practices would inevitably discourage necessary patient care. Thus, like some employers, French Communist leaders were also acting "out of character," withholding their usual support for forceful state action. They would have nothing to do with a national health service, wishing instead to sustain the freedoms of doctors and patients in the private sector.[22] All these positions exemplify how the tensions evoked by cost control measures cut across traditional right-left political cleavages. Meanwhile, a comparably dizzying debate was taking place in the United States.

HMOs and Cost Control in the United States

As in France, when U.S. political leaders addressed the problem of health care inflation, they bemoaned the unwieldy provision of medical care services. Health, Education, and Welfare (HEW) secretary Douglas Coleman complained, "Almost all medical care costs are generated either by a professional decision or by professional acquiescence with a patient's demand....At the root of the medical care cost problem is the fact that most of these decisions are made outside any organizational framework which holds the physician accountable for or even makes him aware...of the economic consequences of the totality of these individual decisions."[23]

President Richard Nixon shared the HEW secretary's frustration. He was joined by members of Congress, including Senator Thomas Eagleton, who told the Blue Cross Association's president, Walter McNerney, that "the present system is all together too cozy a quasi-incestuous relationship" between insurers and providers.[24] Coleman and Eagleton were concerned about physicians' continued use of "usual, customary, and reasonable" billing and about the fact that hospitals charged insurers, including Medicare and Medicaid, their entire costs plus a generous overhead allowance. In neither ambulatory nor inpatient care did there exist sufficient mechanisms by which insurers could monitor medical decision makers, which reformers on both sides of the Atlantic considered a first step toward cost control.

Just as in France, powerful U.S. employers, who were footing much of the nation's health care bill, finally broke with the medical profession and called for change. One analyst explained: "The National Association of Manufacturers, the U.S. Chamber of Commerce, and the Republican leadership were generally allies of the AMA. But concern over escalating costs...[has] made cost containment the major new political strategy in health care...and the business community its principle proponents."[25] As one corporate executive put it, health care needed "'three wonder drugs': (1) real management, (2) a meaningful system of incentives and disincentives, and (3) the opportunity for each consumer to choose the basic medical services he feels he can afford."[26] By 1970, U.S. employers' tolerance for doctors' and hospitals' broad liberties of treatment and billing had clearly reached its limit.

Meanwhile, in Washington, President Nixon faced a formidable political challenge. Senator Edward Kennedy of Massachusetts had launched a far-reaching health care reform initiative with his health security bill. Kennedy called for the creation of a single, national health insurance system to replace Medicare, Medicaid, and private insurance. Physicians and hospitals would remain autonomous providers, private or public as the case may be; to stem inflation, however, Kennedy foresaw a national health care budget. Creation of a global budget for health care spending threatened private practitioners' billing liberties and would have forced hospitals to seek efficiencies in their care. For workers, Kennedy offered universal coverage with no coinsurance payments. It was within this context—employers' frustration with rising health care inflation and

Kennedy's proposal for national health insurance—that health maintenance organizations (HMOs) and managed care in general overtook U.S. health care.

The core idea of HMOs was hardly new. Medical care providers, be they doctors or hospitals, instead of simply billing for services provided, must share responsibility with insurers for their patients' health. Earlier we saw that rural populists and industrial paternalists had both created distinct health care financing and delivery systems built on this idea. In so doing, they had challenged the medical profession's insistence on private-practice liberties. In the 1930s, two dozen general practitioners and specialists, backed by the Oklahoma Farmers' Union, had joined together in a rural medical cooperative under the leadership of Michael Shadid. Physicians accepted capitated payments for the treatment of most ailments and thereby shared financial responsibility for the health and eventual recovery of their patients. On a much larger scale, the western concrete and shipbuilding magnate Henry Kaiser opened the health care facilities he had built specially for his workers to the general public after the Second World War. Kaiser thus created prepaid comprehensive insurance plans that also ran counter to traditional fee-for-service payment and practice liberties. Under Kaiser plans, patients sought care from a Kaiser hospital and its associated group of physicians, most of whom were salaried Kaiser Plan employees.

Kaiser doctors had every incentive to return their patients to health as quickly as possible since, unlike fee-for-service arrangements, additional tests and therapies only increased the plan's costs without bringing added revenues. Moreover, studies indicated that Kaiser practitioners collaborated more closely than disparate private practitioners in their efforts to speed patient recovery. Although Kaiser failed to realize his dream of transforming U.S. medicine, Kaiser plans remained strong and well subscribed in their home regions of California and the Pacific Northwest. Elsewhere, however, they faced immovable opposition from state medical societies, backed by the AMA and supported in state legislatures, which were hostile to Kaiser's use of salaried physicians and its abrogation of traditional fee-for-service arrangements.[27] This opposition, along with the popularity of Blue Cross and Blue Shield plans among union and nonunion workers alike, greatly constrained the expansion of Kaiser and similar early HMOs. But with pressure from employers and Congress mounting, the Nixon White House cast a broad net in its search for initiatives that could solve the "health care crisis," a term Kennedy had successfully transferred to the popular media by 1970.[28]

In February of that year, Nixon aides met with Paul M. Ellwood, a Minneapolis rehabilitation specialist and director of the American Rehabilitation Foundation. Ellwood, a longtime advocate of Kaiser-style comprehensive health plans, presented a particularly transparent case (for laypeople) against the perverse incentives perpetuated by fee-for-service. That system penalized providers whose care resulted in a patient's speedy rehabilitation after, say, orthopedic surgery, and, by paying for additional medical visits, rewarded those that provided ineffective or slow-working therapy.

In other words, Ellwood played the role in the United States that Michel Flamme had played in France. Given the different emphasis (private versus public) that had marked the progress of U.S. and French health care since the 1930s, it is fitting that Flamme was a state planning official and Ellwood a backer of private Kaiser-style health plans. Just as Flamme had dared to publicly criticize wasteful fee-for-service medical practices, Ellwood said aloud in the White House what insurers and providers had understood for a long time. Equally important, Ellwood coined a politically appealing new term for prepaid group practice—*health maintenance organization*.

Within a year, Nixon announced his own "national health strategy" to match Kennedy's. HMOs were at its core. In public, Nixon stressed that traditional medical approaches harbored an "illogical incentive": doctors benefited from illness rather than health. But in a private conversation tape-recorded in the Oval Office just a day before the national presentation of his new strategy, the president expressed skepticism about what his own White House wished to propose. Nixon told his aide John Ehrlichman, "You know I'm not keen on any of these damn medical programs." Ehrlichman, however, prevailed, suggesting the appeal that insurers and employers would find in an HMO strategy:

EHRLICHMAN: This—this is a—

PRESIDENT NIXON: I don't [unclear]—

EHRLICHMAN: —private enterprise one.

PRESIDENT NIXON: Well, that appeals to me.

EHRLICHMAN: Edgar Kaiser is running his Permanente deal for profit. And the reason that he can—the reason he can do it—I had Edgar Kaiser come in—talk to me about this and I went into it in some depth. All the incentives are toward less medical care, because—

PRESIDENT NIXON: [Unclear.]

EHRLICHMAN: —the less care they give them, the more money they make.

PRESIDENT NIXON: Fine. [Unclear.]

EHRLICHMAN: [Unclear] and the incentives run the right way.

PRESIDENT NIXON: Not bad.[29]

What followed is surely one of the most remarkable transformations of a domestic policy idea in U.S. history. Edward Kennedy had been advocating incentives for the creation of prepaid group practices since the late 1960s, but he was only the latest in a long line of Democrats who envisioned capitated payment and group practices as key elements of greater health care equality and efficiency. Since the Committee on the Cost of Medical Care had issued its report in 1932, the Left had viewed prepaid group practice as an attractive and cost-effective alternative to fee-for-service practitioners. Now in the early 1970s, under Nixon's leadership, Republicans, including Governors Ronald Reagan of California and Nelson Rockefeller of New York, effectively repackaged what they had previously criticized as utopian, even subversive, into a cost-conscious solution to the nation's health care crisis. As the sociologist Paul Starr puts it, "They had substituted a rhetoric of rationalization and competition for the older rhetoric of cooperation and mutual protection. The socialized medicine of one era had become the corporate reform of the next."[30]

Initially, the major difference between the Right and the Left on prepaid group practice plans was profit. Specifically, what type of insurers would be eligible for government subsidies to set up HMOs? Democrats advocated government support for nonprofit medical corporations, which would operate prepaid plans for underserved populations. The Health Maintenance Organization Act, which Nixon signed into law in 1973, included attention to medically needy areas, but it also made government subsidies available to for-profit insurers, no matter where they operated. Moreover, it defined HMO so loosely that simple networks of independent physicians or associated hospitals, even if reimbursed on a fee-for-service basis, could qualify. Finally, the HMO Act required all employers of more than twenty-five employees, who already provided a health insurance plan, to also offer an HMO option if it were available in their area. This guaranteed HMOs access to the all-important employment-based health insurance market, which state legislators and medical leaders in many parts of the country had long prevented. In return for government subsidies and freedom from state legislative mandates, HMOs had to employ community rating of their plans. This, government officials hoped, would slow the relentless fragmentation of employment-based health insurance pools wrought by the spread of experience-rated policies.

Despite the federal government's intervention on their behalf, HMOs were slow to catch on in the 1970s. After all, even if the name had changed, the stigma attached to prepaid group practices, which explicitly limited patient choice of doctor and implicitly constrained physicians' clinical freedoms, remained a major stumbling block. Of the 40 million dollars in subsidies that had been appropriated under the 1973 HMO Act, just a little over half had been spent by 1975.[31] After 1976, now under President Jimmy Carter, a Democrat, the federal government responded by waiving HMOs' obligation to community rating and by further loosening the government's definition of comprehensive medical coverage, a requisite criterion to qualify for subsidies.[32]

The easing of eligibility standards, combined with continued health care inflation, finally led to a dramatic rise in the creation and enrollment of HMOs during the 1980s and 1990s. In 1971, 33 HMOs served 3.6 million enrollees. By 1985, 377 HMOs had 16.7 million subscribers, and by century's end nearly 85 percent of workers who enjoyed employment-based coverage were enrolled in an HMO or some form of managed care plan with its origins in the HMO movement—a preferred provider organization (PPO) or point-of-service plan (POS). In short, in less than twenty-five years, the HMO movement begun in the early 1970s had reversed the proportion of enrollees in traditional fee-for-service versus managed care plans.[33]

As one observer of the managed care revolution in U.S. medicine remarked, "Everyone loves HMOs except for two groups...doctors and patients." Even if this remark oversimplified the discontent about managed care restrictions of patient choice and doctors' clinical freedoms, it captured tensions over utilization constraints and medical resources. In particular, a further emphasis on "private enterprise," as John Ehrlichman had put it in his Oval Office briefing of Nixon, raised questions of health care quality and access. Nixon's triumph over Kennedy, and the resulting embrace of greater leeway for private insurers and market forces to control health care costs, were hardly unique to the United States. French leaders also wished to go beyond their 1971 national *convention,* which had transferred a greater share of physician fees to patients. Incoming U.S. president Ronald Reagan pursued a comparable strategy at about the same time.

Promarket Reformers in France and the United States

In 1976, President Valéry Giscard d'Estaing appointed a promarket economist, Raymond Barre, to be prime minister. Like proponents of the managed care movement brewing in the United States, Barre wished to recast the price incentives of French health care. Specifically, Barre viewed higher doctors' fees, to be borne by patients, as a helpful tonic for wasteful consumers of medical services. In the freedom of the marketplace, reasoned Barre, patients should be willing to pay more for physicians who were more experienced, thereby shouldering a greater share of the nation's health care bill based on their own judgment. But Barre's approach faced a serious obstacle.

Not only did most workers obtain their *Sécurité Sociale* health coverage through their workplace (or that of a family member), they also benefited from private supplemental insurance, often through the same employer or professional association. In fact, by the 1970s, mutual societies had been joined in the supplemental insurance business by dozens of for-profit companies. In 1980, 69 percent of the population enjoyed some sort of health insurance coverage above and beyond *Sécurité Sociale*, a proportion that was increasing rapidly and would reach 86 percent by 2000.[34]

If Prime Minister Barre wished to simultaneously slow *Sécurité Sociale* spending and health care inflation by trimming demand for medical care services, he had to prevent supplemental insurers from picking up the medical bills that *Sécurité Sociale* refused to cover. Otherwise, patients and doctors could merrily continue their health care utilization habits without regard for price. This led Barre in 1979 to propose that patients be required to pay no less than 5 percent of their doctor bills from their own pockets. The response was swift and overwhelming. Doctors, unions, and private insurers pummeled the proposal, forcing Barre into a hasty retreat.

Ronald Reagan experienced a comparable defeat in the early years of his presidency. Like their counterparts in France's finance ministry, economists at the U.S. Treasury wished to induce the spread of *less* comprehensive health insurance. Less comprehensive policies would have forced patients to pay more out-of-pocket expenses, thereby reducing demand for medical care, and in theory, slowing inflation. Unlike in France, U.S. government officials shied away from seeking to outlaw supplemental insurance that completely eliminated patient cost. Instead, in 1982, Ronald Reagan proposed a cap on the tax deductibility of health insurance premiums, which would have raised the cost of comprehensive health coverage for both employers and workers, since they would have had to pay the portion of their premium exceeding 150 dollars per month from after-tax dollars. Equally important, the 150-dollar maximum for tax deductibility would increase only with the consumer price index, not at the much higher health care inflation rate. In turn, some of the government's increased tax revenues would have been rebated to employers as an incentive to offer their workers *less* comprehensive medical insurance plans.[35]

Like Barre, Reagan wanted to increase patients' expenses and thereby sensitize them to the price of medical care. Both leaders wished to force their fellow citizens to trim their habits of unnecessary doctor visits and medical procedures. But both proposals would have created substantial inequities between the healthy and the chronically ill. Forced to seek serious medical care more often, the sick would have faced higher medical care expenditures, either through greater out-of-pocket expenditures, higher insurance premiums, or both. Also, physicians quickly pointed out that patients were not sufficiently knowledgeable consumers. They often mistook the early symptoms of a major malady, which could be treated at relatively little expense if caught early, for a minor ailment. Under these circumstances, discouraging patients from seeking care through higher out-of-pocket expenses could result in greater patient suffering and much higher health care expenditures for patients and insurers in the long run.

Like Barre two years earlier, Reagan received a withering response to his proposal from across the political spectrum, including employers and his fellow Republicans. Robert Packwood, the Republican chair of the Senate Finance Committee, dismissed the proposal but took time to teach a short history lesson to White House officials. "One reason we do not have any significant demand for national health insurance in this country among those who are employed is because their employers are paying for their benefits.... I hate to see us nibble at [that system.]"[36] On both sides of the Atlantic, then, promarket reformers ran up against their nation's health care history. Driven back as they were from initiatives that would have directly increased patients' costs, political leaders in France and the United States refocused their attention on health care's supply side, namely, physician services and hospital reimbursement.

Dividing France's Doctors

In 1980, *Sécurité Sociale* reported that the monitoring of physician treatment practices, as agreed on under the national *convention* of 1971, was failing to have the desired effect of constraining the utilization of medical services. What is more, even though the government had instituted tighter restrictions on the number of students entering medical school under its so-called *numerus clausus* powers over medical education, the number of doctors continued to rise and with it the demand for medical services. Between 1955 and 1979, France witnessed a 120 percent rise in the number of practicing physicians. Although salaried positions had also increased, most doctors remained attached to their fee-for-service practices. In 1979, fully 71 percent of practitioners maintained private offices and nearly 40 percent devoted themselves full time to fee-for-service medicine; the remaining 31 percent worked for hospitals or in other salaried positions but kept a substantial private-patient clientele. Moreover, the number of private practitioners was projected to increase another 26 percent by 1985, from 78,250 to 98,850.

Thus, when the national *convention* that governed doctors' fees came up for renewal in 1980, Prime Minister Barre announced the creation of a national health care budget, which, by its very definition, indicated his intent to curb physicians' medical decision making and thereby *Sécurité Sociale* health care spending. Spending increases were limited to 12 percent per year, substantially more than the current rate of consumer inflation but far below the 16.5 percent that analysts predicted for health care.

The CSMF, which represented 45 percent of doctors, responded with a one-day strike (excluding urgent and emergency care) to protest Barre's proposal. Just over half the French population voiced support for physicians. Days after the strike, *Panorama du Médecin*, a medical journal, commissioned an independent polling organization to query public opinion. Pollsters asked: "If more stringent controls meant that doctors had to limit prescriptions, tests, appointments, etc., what would you say?" Respondents were provided with three options. Twenty-six percent responded that "it's normal because health care costs too much"; 51 percent said, "it's inappropriate because health care should not have a price." And 18 percent answered: "That's my doctor's problem, not mine."[37]

With popular opinion tending to support doctors, CSMF leaders refused negotiations. Barre then turned to the much smaller medical *syndicat*, the Fédération des Médecins de France (FMF), which could claim only 15 percent of medical professionals as members. The law required that *Sécurité Sociale* and the government reach a negotiated settlement with physicians but did not define exactly what that meant. This permitted Barre to pursue the politically precarious, albeit legal, strategy of trying to reach an agreement with the FMF. Sticking by his plans for a national health care budget, Barre banked on his promarket measures to attract the conservative FMF to the negotiating table. The tactic worked. In exchange for greater billing freedoms for more doctors, the FMF signed a new national *convention* in 1980.

Both parties agreed that if an increased supply of doctors had resulted in more medical services sold, that is, if supply had actually created its own demand, thereby forcing up expenditures, then the solution must be, at least in part, to permit more doctors to charge more than standard fees. Rising prices could stem demand and help relieve *Sécurité Sociale* of its financial woes. Even if patients had supplemental insurance, Barre reasoned, the price of comprehensive policies that left patients with no out-of-pocket expenses would rise as insurers sought protection from greater liabilities. So-called balance-billing policies, which reimbursed patients based solely on standard *convention* fees, not actual physician charges, would quickly replace comprehensive supplemental insurance. The result would be a dampening of demand and a reduction in health care utilization. This, of course, was the theory. Exactly what the government, *Sécurité Sociale*, and the FMF agreed to warrants a full explanation since it marked a major turning point in French health care, comparable to the opening of the managed care era in the United States.

After 1980, French doctors could choose one of three *sectors* of practice. Those who selected Sector 1 agreed to abide by standard *convention* fees except in particularly difficult cases, under which they could seek a special dispensation. Physicians who, under the 1971 *convention,* already enjoyed waivers to exceed standard fees because of their exceptional experience or training could continue to do so, but no more such waivers would be granted. This meant that new doctors entering the profession who wanted to exercise the freedom to bill as they wished had no choice but to join Sector 2.

A Sector 2 physician determined her own fees, but her patients were reimbursed based on the standard (Sector 1) fee and had to make up the difference from out-of-pocket funds or supplemental insurance, as the case may be. To prevent a mass exodus of physicians to Sector 2, the government granted substantial tax breaks and *Sécurité Sociale* retirement, health, and disability benefits to those who remained in Sector 1. Lastly, the *convention* recognized a third group of practitioners, Sector 3, most of whom ran "boutique" allopathic or alternative medical practices (for example, acupuncture or homeopathy) and wished as little connection with *Sécurité Sociale* as possible. Sector 3 patients received only nominal reimbursements of their medical fees from *Sécurité Sociale.*

All of France's unions except the Force Ouvrière joined CSMF leaders in opposing the new *convention.* CSMF president Jacques Monier predicted that "the new liberties of some will be paid for by the imprisonment of others." Monier's critique was double-edged. He believed that the creation of Sector 2 would propagate "a medicine for the rich and a medicine for the poor" and also foresaw the eventual impoverishment of doctors who remained in Sector 1 without fee waivers. Most of these, as it turned out, were general practitioners.[38] In fact, of the nearly 12 percent of doctors who already claimed fee waivers under Sector 1, the vast majority (80 percent) were specialists. Specialists also dominated among the 7.5 percent of physicians who immediately declared their practices under Sector 2.[39]

Physician Declarations June 1981

Sector 1	91.4%
with 1971 fee waiver	11.7%
without fee waiver	79.7%
Sector 2	7.5%
Sector 3	1.1%

Although Prime Minister Barre and President Giscard d'Estaing had defied the political odds by successfully concluding a new *convention* with the minority FMF, they found themselves on the defensive in public. Sixty-one percent of those polled selected the term "shameful" to describe the creation of Sector 2 exclusively for doctors who wished more fee-setting liberty. The polls were bad news for Giscard d'Estaing, who faced a tough reelection challenge from the Socialist François Mitterrand in the 1981 presidential contest. Even more troublesome for the president and his "promarket" prime minister was that half their own supporters, who hailed from center and center-right parties, also disliked the creation of Sector 2. Nonetheless, with the signature of the minority FMF, the new *convention* became law in June 1980, and CSMF doctors were forced to break off their protests and abide by its provisions. The presidential election followed eleven months later. For the first time in decades, doctors voted in large numbers for a leftist presidential candidate, François Mitterrand, helping him to handily defeat the incumbent, Giscard d'Estaing, and to sweep the legislative elections.

The alignment of the leading physicians' association, the CSMF, with the Socialists in the battle over the 1980 *convention* marked a shift in France's health care politics.[40] Recriminations over binding fee schedules, first enforced in 1960, had subsided. Most doctors were accustomed to and even supported the idea of a national *convention*, especially if it included the possibility of case-specific or experience-based fee waivers, which had been granted in 1971. But the creation of Sector 2 appeared to threaten the *convention* system itself. It undermined hard-won compromises between physicians and the state, which had been the hallmark of French health care since 1930, and exacerbated the split between general practitioners and specialists. Like the U.S. government's boost to HMOs in the 1970s, the division of France's doctors into distinct sectors set the stage for more cost shifting to patients and the adoption of managed care techniques in France.

The Fall of the American Medical Association

At first blush, it would appear that the division of French physicians between backers of the CSMF and its rival, the conservative FMF, put France's doctors at a disadvantage compared to their U.S. counterparts. The FMF's willingness to negotiate a new *convention* in 1980 is a case in point. It shattered any hope that CSMF leaders might have had in creating a united front against the government and *Sécurité Sociale*. As long as Prime Minister Barre had the FMF as a willing partner, the opposition of other doctors, even if they represented a majority of the profession, was doomed in advance. The AMA suffered no comparable rivalry in its representation of U.S. doctors.[41]

Yet the vaunted unity of the U.S. medical profession failed to prevent its members from enduring major setbacks during the 1980s. First, the AMA experienced a humiliating defeat when it sought to protect billing freedoms for Medicare patients. Then, with the spread of managed care insurers during the 1990s, U.S. physicians were often subject to financial sanctions and rewards on the basis of their once sacredly independent medical decision making.

AMA president Joseph Boyle had forewarned his colleagues of a brewing fight over Medicare billing in a July 1983 National Press Club speech: "Governments at all levels are placing absolute limits on the dollars that they will spend on care...attempting to prevent individuals from seeking and receiving care even if they can pay for it out of their own resources."[42] Boyle's remark sounded a lot like CSMF president Jacques Monier's objection to his government's announcement of a national health care budget three years earlier. When Medicare was created in 1965, lawmakers had eschewed the French model whereby physicians negotiated fee schedules with the public insurer. As the health care economist Rashi Fein points out, "The Medicare compromise [of 1965] was that the program was not to be used to alter the structure of our health care delivery system. Medicare was to be a neutral conduit for dollars."[43]

That was all well and good when dollars were plentiful and medical care less expensive. In its early years, physicians generally accepted what Medicare termed "assignment." The government determined assignment fees by examining the usual and customary charge of the doctor in question, her charge in the particular case, as well as the price for the same procedure in the surrounding community. As Medicare became more intent on controlling health care expenditures after 1970, doctors began to complain about a lag between their rising customary charges and Medicare's assignment fees. But nothing prevented a doctor from refusing assignment and charging Medicare patients whatever she wished. In fact, about half of all Medicare claims in 1982 rejected assignment. In such cases, the patient paid her physician directly and then applied for a partial reimbursement directly from Medicare. A U.S. doctor who rejected assignment, then, was like a French doctor who, under the *convention* of 1980, declared her practice under Sector 2 and charged *Sécurité Sociale* patients what she wished, leaving them with greater out-of-pocket and/or supplemental insurance costs.

What outraged AMA president Boyle was government plans to force U.S. physicians to declare themselves in this or that sector with regard to Medicare patients, *à la française*. That is, either a doctor pledged to accept assignment for all Medicare patients or she declared her practice nonparticipating. Doctors who committed themselves to assignment were promised faster payment and the listing of their practices in Medicare directories. Moreover, the government offered assurances to participating doctors that, when budget circumstances permitted, their requests for increased assignment fees would be granted before those of their colleagues who had refused to participate. Not only that, nonparticipating physicians who dared to raise fees from what they had charged between April and June 1984 faced fines of two thousand dollars for each and every procedure for which they hiked their fees, as well as the possibility of being barred from treating Medicare patients altogether.

In their unsuccessful attempt to stop enactment of the mandate, AMA lobbyists descended on Capitol Hill. Executive vice president James Sammons urged members of Congress to reject compulsory measures. Instead, he pledged that "the AMA will ask physicians to refrain from passing on additional costs to their elderly patients."[44] But like French medical leaders, who had promised that their members would avoid significant fee hikes for *Sécurité Sociale* beneficiaries in the 1950s, the AMA wielded no surefire way to control individual practitioners' fees. U.S. political leaders thus ultimately ignored the AMA's appeals for many of the same reasons that the French government finally adopted binding fee schedules. Their political accountability to beneficiaries proved more important than their vulnerability to a major professional association.

What is striking about the Medicare assignment episode is its departure from the "promarket" initiatives of the early Reagan years. Medicare fee freezes and civil penalties for doctors who violated them could hardly be defined as "taking advantage of market forces." But where Medicare had resorted to traditional regulatory methods to hold down costs, HMOs created a raft of novel financial incentives to divorce physicians and patients from the liberties they had long enjoyed under fee-for-service health insurance plans.

Beginning in the 1980s, the AMA's political muscle failed to protect physicians' professional sovereignty in the face of an unprecedented reorganization of U.S. medicine by new managed care corporations. Apart from a historical aversion to government intervention, which was of little help under the circumstances, medical leaders had no alternative unifying vision that could effectively combat the encroachment of insurers into clinical decision making. In fact, many physicians joined the managed care movement by founding HMOs themselves or signing on as medical specialty executives. In contrast to France, in the United States a legal vacuum regarding patient rights and physician liberties granted the new health care corporations, which often combined insurer and provider, with tremendous leeway to remake medicine.

Of course, reformers who supported the growth of managed care viewed health care not as a vacuum but as an exciting new for-profit industry where entrepreneurship and innovation could solve the problems of spiraling costs, limited access, and poor quality. Even the national directors of Blue Cross and Blue Shield, early proponents and stalwart defenders of fee-for-service nonprofit health insurance, voted in 1994 to allow its regional plans to develop for-profit HMOs.[45] The florescence of managed care severely reduced the medical sovereignty of U.S. physicians when compared with their French colleagues. This development was on the same scale as professional turning points earlier in the century.

In 1930, French doctors had reached a compromise with state officials that permitted the country's first national health insurance program for industrial workers. Known as the "medical charter," it defined private fee-for-service practice, physicians' clinical freedoms, and patient choice as indispensable to quality health care. Through war, defeat, German occupation, and three constitutions, the charter remained a salient political rallying point to which doctors and patients turned when threatened with government or private insurers' restrictions on patient choice or physician freedoms. Whenever medical sovereignty was threatened, doctors labeled the offending proposals "assembly-line medicine" and "health care ration-ing" to invoke its industrial and impersonal nature. Such rhetoric can still be heard today from medical leaders who wish to recall past victories and thereby fortify present protections for autonomous private practitioners. To be sure, private-practice freedoms have been curtailed since their heyday mid-century, and aspects of managed care have been adopted by *Sécurité Sociale*. Also, French physicians, on average, do not enjoy nearly the in-comes of their U.S. counterparts.[46] But on questions of professional sov-ereignty, U.S. physicians, in stark contrast to French doctors, beat a hasty retreat from the ideals of private-practice medicine, ideals to which both had sworn allegiance since the 1920s. The Americans surrendered their exclusive control over medical decision making, fee-for-service, and pa-tient choice when they came face-to-face with determined insurers' efforts to trim costs.[47]

When AMA leader Morris Fishbein asked in 1934, "Shall the doctor or the insurance adjuster say how long the patient is to lie in bed after an operation for appendicitis?" he did so only rhetorically.[48] None of his colleagues would have pleaded the part of the insurer. And if Fishbein had asked why not, he would have heard a chorus, "because a patient's health has no price and that's all the insurance adjuster cares about." By 1982, however, 58 percent of U.S. doctors considered cost to be the main problem facing medicine, up from 44 percent only a year before. Doctors were not alone. After 1977, cost steadily outstripped quality of care and access as the primary concern of the general public.[49] In November 1983, the AMA's Council on Medical Service formally recommended that the as-sociation discontinue its long-standing policy of supporting doctors' use of "usual, customary, and reasonable" billing. According to the council, the AMA had no choice. More and more insurers were refusing to pay such charges, which left patients with the impression that their doctors' fees were somehow "unreasonable."[50] And the change was not just about language. Increasing numbers of doctors were signing contracts for capi-tated compensation or were accepting salaried positions with managed care providers.

These arrangements are varied and complex. But their overriding trait is that a physician (or group of physicians) accepts a measure of risk and stands to reap rewards based on the level of medical services their patients use. This risk/reward dynamic motivates managed care's focus on preventive medicine. After all, an ailment avoided is an ailment for which the practitioner does not have to provide care, thereby conserving resources. It also explains why many early managed care providers embraced the term *health maintenance*. Obviously, healthy subscribers cost the provider little. Even the treatment of chronically ill patients is less expensive when their conditions are monitored and controlled than when the patient episodically seeks major (and costly) interventions.[51]

The earliest HMOs generally owned medical care facilities and employed primary care physicians and specialists who provided both inpatient and ambulatory care directly to subscribers. Strictly speaking, this is the Kaiser model. The 1980s, however, witnessed the growth of myriad variations on this arrangement. Group and network HMOs sometimes own no medical facilities but simply contract with organizations, such as hospitals or clinics, that do. Another model is the independent practice association (IPA) whereby·the HMO contracts with an IPA, which is free to purchase medical services from physicians, paying them either by capitation or under fee-for-service arrangements. The popular preferred provider organization (PPO) is a hybrid between an IPA and traditional health insurance. Enrollees may seek care from a limited number of network physicians, so-called preferred providers, and pay out of pocket only a low co-payment. If a patient goes outside the network to a physician of her choice, she faces a substantial coinsurance fee, usually 30 to 40 percent of billed services. The additional cost incurred by the patient who leaves the PPO network stems from the absence of the risk/reward dynamic that is the hallmark of managed care.[52]

Regardless of the managed care model, medical care providers and physicians are subject to incentives that curb the use of health care services. Again, the incentives are as varied as the models and contracts negotiated between providers, physicians, and managed care insurers. An HMO-employed primary care physician who exceeds target referral rates to specialists often faces an annual salary deduction that has been agreed on in advance. A PPO network physician who orders costly diagnostic testing that surpasses agreed-on utilization rates faces the possibility that the managed care insurer may not renew her contract. Conversely, physicians who meet or undercut utilization rates are often rewarded through profit sharing and/or substantial salary bonuses. As the health care legal scholar Marc Rodwin explains, "One suspects that doctors contracting with or employed by an HMO will, over time, develop an intuitive sense of what style of medical practice best serves their interest. Their practice style will reflect the incentives offered by the HMOs."[53]

Studies of quality under managed care are, according to a leading health care economist, "decidedly ambiguous." Managed care did play a major role in slowing overall health care expenditures, at least until the mid-1990s, when health care inflation reemerged.[54] But there is little doubt that the spread of managed care changed what it meant to be a doctor. During the 1980s, the *Journal of the American Medical Association* was strewn with laments about doctors' newfound dilemmas between, as one contributor put it, "the necessity of limiting costs... [and] the fear of legal liability.... The medical profession must realize that in light of fiscal constraints, an individual physician... may no longer be able to be an unbiased patient advocate."[55]

What AMA leader Morris Fishbein had most feared in 1934, that insurers would oversee physicians in the examining room, had indeed come to pass by 1984. Legal sanctions to guard patients from dangerous risk/reward arrangements and conflicts of interest developed only slowly and inconsistently, and addressed only the most egregious cases. All the AMA could do, as its president shrilly told its members, was to "dig in our heels and say, 'Enough!'"[56] But the moment for such resistance had long passed. Political leaders, employers, and workers, who were paying the bills, had lost their reverence for doctors' professional sovereignty and no longer feared the AMA's political might. Or if they did, they feared far more the skyrocketing cost of health care.[57] In 1994, the chairman of the AMA's board of trustees, Lonnie Bristow, unknowingly echoed Morris Fishbein's 1934 injunction against insurers. Bristow demanded to know: "Who is going to decide what kind of care patients get? Patients? Their physicians? Or will insurance companies and giant corporations take the examining room, pushing patients aside?"[58] Unfortunately for U.S. doctors, the second time they appeared, these questions had lost so much of their rhetorical edge that even doctors were unsure of the answer.

While some physicians had joined or created HMOs, others had gone to the other extreme. In February 1994, David G. Murray, chairman of the conservative American College of Surgeons, which had long opposed national health insurance, testified before a congressional subcommittee *in favor* of expanding Medicare to achieve universal coverage. Murray reported that his organization's about-face had come "out of frustration with insurer-run managed-care plans and a desire to bring about reforms that permit patients to select the physician or surgeon of their choice."[59] Clearly, some U.S. doctors now wished to revisit their earlier opposition to public health insurance and to take advantage of statutory protections of their clinical freedoms and fee-for-service practices. In short, they wished to make the choice that French physicians had made in 1930.

Although the growth of large managed care corporations was made possible by a Nixon White House in search of a health care strategy, the insurers themselves remained in the private sector. This allowed the new health care corporations a nearly unrestricted gambit to restrain health care liberties previously regarded as sacred across the political spectrum. By 2003, HMO and PPO plans together boasted 185 million enrollees, that is, 64 percent of the total population and 74 percent of those who possessed health insurance, a truly remarkable feat. Managed care insurers had simultaneously constrained patients' free choice of doctor and imposed clinical practice norms on physicians. Even more remarkably, surprisingly few referred to managed care as health care rationing, which, for historical reasons, Americans usually associated only with the government. This was perhaps managed care's greatest victory.

As the search for cost control spread, hospitals could not be overlooked. In this area, the United States and France adopted similar approaches to stem the financial hemorrhaging of their public insurance programs.

8

HOSPITALS AND THE DIFFICULT ART OF HEALTH CARE REFORM, 1980–PRESENT

Social systems are never saved by true believers, the virtues
appropriate to going down with the ship rarely being suitable
to the arts of navigation.

ROBERT SKIDELSKY on social reformers

Hospitals underwent a substantial transformation during
the twentieth century. French hospitals, in particular, had a history of religious charity care that dated back several centuries, usually under the
auspices of a Catholic diocese. Successive republican governments of the
nineteenth century, however, transferred hospital control to public authorities. But the state's displacement of religious authority remained deeply
unsatisfying to the unions and employers that dominated *Sécurité Sociale*
governing boards after 1945. They believed that, since workers and employers essentially paid for hospitals through payroll levies, they should
have a corresponding influence in their management.

"We just don't understand why," complained a leading *Sécurité Sociale*
official in 1954, "*Sécurité Sociale* devotes a significant portion of its resources to hospitals but is not commensurately involved in the problems
raised by hospitalization, hospital transformation, and new conceptions of
hospitals." Government officials could not entirely ignore *Sécurité Sociale*
demands, but Ministry of Health officials believed that hospital management had to be entrusted to specially trained administrators, not union
leaders.[1] This policy was reinforced shortly after the creation of France's
Fifth Republic and the election of Charles de Gaulle as its first president
in 1958.

In that year, the government pushed through changes that strengthened the minister of health's control of hospitals at the expense of both *Sécurité Sociale* and local authorities. The reform paired regional hospitals with medical schools. The resulting university medical complexes were endowed with full-time clinical faculty, who were integrated into hospital management. The remaining public hospitals also acquired full-time salaried physicians in certain specialties while protecting the hospital practice privileges of community physicians. Finally, the reform brought the capital investments of all hospitals, public and private, under government supervision. In 1970, the Ministry of Health further tightened criteria for capital expansions, drawing up a medical map (*carte sanitaire*) through which the government hoped to avoid wasteful expenditures on excess beds and redundant technologies. Despite the heavy hand of the state, private nonprofit and for-profit hospitals continued to flourish, accounting for one-third of all beds and half of those devoted to obstetrics and surgery.[2]

The United States' postwar hospital expansion paralleled the French in scope, but it protected rather than diminished local control, and slowed rather than spurred a rationalization of hospital expansion. Between 1946 and 1975 the Hill-Burton Act allocated federal funds for hospital construction based on local and state criteria. No state could be denied Hill-Burton monies unless it had more than 4.5 hospital beds per thousand residents, a generous allotment even by care standards of the day, which stressed postsurgical bed rest rather than today's emphasis on early ambulation. (In 2004, the United States possessed 2.8 acute care beds per thousand residents, compared with France's 3.8.)[3] Between 1947 and 1971, Hill-Burton disbursed 3.7 billion dollars and contributed to 30 percent of all projects nationwide. Over time, 4.5 hospital beds per thousand residents became a target instead of a ceiling, as originally intended, thereby exacerbating supply-driven health care inflation in subsequent decades. Moreover, although many rural communities in dire need acquired facilities thanks to Hill-Burton, the law failed to help the most needy because it required all grantees to demonstrate the future financial viability of their projects, a criterion that excluded many of the poorest communities in the country. Hill-Burton also fell short in its goal of creating the regional health networks its backers had promised. After grants were awarded, the law required no collaboration between facilities, which might have led to earlier improvements in hospital productivity.[4]

In light of this contrast, one might suppose that France's far more state-centered postwar hospital expansion would continue to diverge from its

U.S. counterpart. Just as U.S. and French medical leaders' different inter-war decisions on compulsory medical insurance set in motion a seemingly irreversible momentum toward contrasting approaches to health security (private versus public), hospitals too, the supposition goes, would continue to become more diverse. But the truth is far more interesting and surprising.

In the early 1980s, as both nations searched for ways to control rising hospital expenditures, President François Mitterrand embraced a new and singularly U.S. invention: prospective payment for hospital services based on diagnosis related groups (DRGs). At the time, neither Medicare, which paid for services on a cost-plus basis, nor *Sécurité Sociale*, which was experimenting with global hospital budgets, had found an effective way to induce cost savings from hospital administrators. In both countries, the longer patients stayed in hospital, the larger the bill and the greater the hospital's income.[5]

By using DRGs, an insurer could turn the tables. Instead of paying after the fact for whatever services were provided, the insurer fixed prices in advance for hospital treatment of specific diagnoses; hence the term diagnosis related group. In short, hospitals now had products called DRGs whose prices were set by the public insurer. If they produced a DRG, whether a kidney transplant or treatment for a concussion, for less than the going price, the hospital kept the difference.

Ironically, this convergence in U.S. and French hospitals came from leaders with opposing ideologies. France's adoption of DRGs grew directly out of the 1981 election of Socialist president François Mitterrand, who promised to expand social welfare programs. As the most important change in French presidential leadership since de Gaulle's election in 1958, Mitterrand's administration swept from their posts entrenched civil servants who might have blocked or sabotaged major policy reorientations. Jean de Kervasdoué, who became undersecretary for hospitals at the Ministry of Health under Mitterrand, had for some time been following the work to improve hospital efficiency conducted by Yale University researchers Robert Fetter and John Thompson. Indeed, France's DRG pilot studies in 1982 marked the first such testing outside the United States, but Socialist losses in parliamentary elections in 1986 slowed full-fledged implementation until the mid-1990s.[6] In the United States, DRGs also owed their implementation to a newly elected president, Ronald Reagan. But in contrast to Mitterrand, Reagan was a conservative who promised an era of deregulation and cutbacks in the U.S. welfare state. Did Mitterrand's embrace of DRGs mean that France had renounced its state-directed hospital policy? Hardly.

The Franco-American entente over DRGs was technocratic rather than ideological. To the extent that ideology did play a role, the Americans were the ones doing the renouncing. After all, prospective hospital payment and more stringent accountability were taken up first by Medicare, not by private insurers. Indeed, it is unlikely that market forces could have produced DRGs' all-important consistency. Medicare followed its implementation of DRGs with a physician fee schedule based on the same idea. Resource-based relative value scales (RBRVS) estimated the training, time, and skill necessary for specific procedures and paid doctors accordingly. A former U.S. government health care official explains, "Medicare provided the first organized national attempt to address the issue of utilization...because Medicare was a single large national program with much at stake while other payers were smaller and fragmented and each had less to gain from control efforts."[7]

Evidence suggests that DRGs' national price controls could be even more effective than private insurers at constraining inpatient costs. Between 1985 and 1990, Medicare's hospital expenditures fell from 28.9 to 26.1 percent of total national hospital outlays. What is more, between 1984 and 1992, even though Medicare is responsible for the sickest and most elderly patients, its per capita spending grew less rapidly than private insurers' for medical services covered by both.[8] In fact, the first private insurers—all Blue Cross–Blue Shield—to follow Medicare in implementing prospective hospital payment in 1985 hailed from states where their low market shares had prevented them from obtaining significant discounts from hospitals. Only national government action impelled widespread hospital efficiency.[9] If private insurers had achieved cost savings in ambulatory care by creating HMOs, the United States' public insurer for the elderly, Medicare, had achieved an equally impressive feat in the hospital sector. Or had it?

As a national health insurer, France's *Sécurité Sociale* employed DRGs to determine global hospital budgets, not necessarily to calculate individual patient bills. By using DRGs while at the same time developing the country's broader medical information system, the health ministry and *Sécurité Sociale* could allocate health care resources more efficiently and with less political risk. In no small measure, Ministry of Health officials continued to rely on the Yale University Health Services Management Group. In the end, however, French authorities succeeded in creating a specifically French case mix, known as *groupes homogènes de malades* (homogeneous patient groups, or GHMs).[10]

Since 1998, all French hospitals and clinics of any kind—public, private for-profit, or nonprofit—have been required to use GHMs to manage resources, quality of care, and epidemiological studies. Hospital revenues are determined by a mix of their GHM production, global budgeting, and the local circumstances that affect medical care costs.[11] To be sure, the implementation of prospective hospital payment in France was not without difficulties. Political wrangling and doctors' resistance repeatedly interrupted implementation, and inadequate information technology slowed their effectiveness and spread.[12] Ultimately, however, the comprehensive scope of GHM implementation in France, alongside the country's similarly comprehensive *conventions* governing ambulatory care, helped the country avoid pitfalls experienced in the United States.

Because of the United States' more fragmented health care system, DRGs may have actually spurred medical inflation rather than slowing it. Medicare's DRGs and their inevitable spin-offs among private insurers affected only inpatient hospital charges. This caused more expensive growth elsewhere. Indeed, policy analysts, who liken the U.S. health care system to a balloon, point to DRGs as a case in point. When one part is squeezed, they note, it bulges in another. By the mid-1990s, skeptics such as the health economist Uwe Reinhardt were questioning the systemic wisdom of DRGs and managed care insurers' subsequent efforts to tighten the noose around hospital stays. Yes, between 1980 and 1993 hospital stays fell by 36 percent, but real (inflation-adjusted) per capita spending on inpatient care rose nearly 53 percent, and real spending on all health services rose by more than 87 percent. In other words, exclaimed Reinhardt, while "the United States was busily emptying its hospitals in the name of cost control, total national health spending actually shot up from 8.9 percent of GDP in 1980 to more than 13.6 percent in 1993."[13]

Managed care insurers and Medicare authorities had become so obsessed by the mantra, "hospitals are very expensive places," that they had unwittingly fostered even more expensive alternatives. For example, because of tight prospective payment schemes, hospitals drastically trimmed convalescent care for postsurgical patients, even though, from a systemic perspective, it remained a relatively cost-effective solution. Instead, a hospital could realize more revenue by discharging the patient to its own subacute care facility, which, in contrast to the hospital, Medicare paid for on a generous cost-plus basis. Alternatively, a patient could be sent home, where an itinerant physical therapist (PT) would provide additional care but at a high per diem rate.[14] Again, from a systemic perspective, a hospital staff PT could have provided rehabilitative care less expensively if only the patient's stay in the hospital had been extended by a few more days, as it would have been in France. Indeed, this helps us understand why France can possess 3.8 hospital beds per thousand residents, provide the same quality of care, and spend far less than the United States, with its 2.8 beds per thousand residents.

Despite France's entrenched state hospital bureaucracies, its implementation of DRGs proved more salutary to the system as a whole because of prohibitions on creating relatively inefficient alternatives to ancillary outpatient and ambulatory care services that would have fallen outside prospective pricing. Medicare and private insurers, conversely, in pursuing their own ends, led U.S. health care into a reform cul-de-sac. As Reinhardt observes, "Techniques that may look efficient from the worm's-eye view of a particular insurer paying for the management of a particular episode of illness actually may be quite inefficient from the more systemic bird's eye view of society."[15] Demographic and technological change notwithstanding, the dramatic growth in the U.S. home health care business, the expansion of subacute care facilities, and the proliferation of outpatient surgery centers became vitally linked to a mind-set that blindly insisted that hospital stays be avoided.

This mind-set imploded in the mid-1990s, when states across the country passed legislation that stopped insurers from forcing new mothers and their babies to be discharged within twenty-four hours of a conventional birth and forty-eight hours after a Cesarean section, often over the objections of their physicians. In signing into law New Jersey's legislation, which granted new mothers and babies another day of convalescence, Republican governor Christine Todd Whitman remarked that insurers needed a dose of "common sense."[16] The comparison between the U.S. and French experiences with cost control in the hospital sector indicates that more centralized health care planning, far from hindering "commonsense" outcomes, can sometimes be vital to their realization.

Médecine à Deux Vitesses (Two-Class Health Care)

Although France's hospital sector escaped some of the controversies that befell its U.S. counterpart, this did not head off a larger crisis in French health care. Like Americans, the French had made little headway in solving the great dilemma of cost control. By 1991, a seemingly inexhaustible demand for ever-better and ever more expensive medical care, combined with broad provider and patient freedoms, had propelled health care spending to 9.1 percent of the GDP. French health care was now the third most expensive in the world, behind the United States (13.4 percent) and Canada (10.0 percent, expressed as a percentage of national income). Voters demanded that the government reduce *Sécurité Sociale* deficits, whose growth was unsustainable. But whenever political leaders tried to do so, they faced firestorms of public protest. Reform of *Sécurité Sociale*, especially its health care component, had become, as pundits often say of Social Security in the United States, a "third rail." Leaders who touched it risked political suicide.

By far the safest way for a French political leader to broach the subject was to raise fears of United States–style health care taking hold in France. A 1990 *Le Monde* editorial by Béatrice Majnoni d'Intignano, an advisor to Prime Minister Michel Rocard, asked: "American health care has, in effect, sounded the alarm: laissez-faire without restriction, is ultracostly. Americans spend more than two thousand dollars per person per year—[we spend] thirteen hundred dollars in France. For whites, their life expectancy is the same as ours. For blacks, it's five years less, and 37 million Americans are uncovered. Is there a better example of *la médecine à deux vitesses* than this temple of private-practice medical liberties?"[17] When Minister of Social Affairs René Teulade insisted in 1992 that medical expenditures simply had to be controlled, he too raised the specter of a United States–style two-class health care system. Concluding an interview with *Le Monde*, Teulade posed a rhetorical question, whose answer in most readers' minds he could be sure of. "And if we don't succeed at saving our system, we'll be headed straight for the American system. Do we really want a third of the population outside the health care system?"[18]

Inaccuracies aside, the larger importance of these remarks was their motive.[19] The French had long viewed their health care system as "the best in the world," not just for its quality but also for its patient choice and autonomous practitioners who were free to prescribe as they wished.[20] Yet now that other revered republican principle, *equality*, appeared to be at risk. In short, the French public sensed the country was headed in the wrong direction on health care, that they were going backward (toward the United States) on France's promise of universal access to quality care.[21]

The fear was not unfounded. A 1993 law expanded the number of ambulatory treatments for which patients face co-payments of 30 percent, a move that fell hardest on those least able to afford it. Even more troubling, unprecedented numbers of physicians had declared their practices in Sector 2, which permitted them to exceed standard fees. In certain regions it had become impossible to find care from a physician who charged standard *Sécurité Sociale* prices. Together with the 3.8 percent of older physicians who retained fee waivers from the 1970s, by 1991 nearly 30 percent of France's doctors no longer abided by *convention* fees, up from 19.5 percent in 1980. On average, these physicians' charges exceeded standard fees by 25 percent, resulting in a near doubling of total receipts surpassing *convention* rates since 1980 (from 4.9 to 9 percent). Not surprisingly, specialists dominated Sector 2 by a ratio of four to one.[22]

Faced with a growing crisis of confidence, government and *Sécurité Sociale* leaders insisted that further admissions to Sector 2 be frozen. This, in turn, provoked a three-sided conflict within the medical profession. Primary care physicians, now united in a new organization, Médecins Généralistes de France (MG-France) sought the abolition of Sector 2 altogether. They rightly viewed its existence as a brake on standard *convention* fees. Meanwhile, within the still-dominant Confédération des Syndicats Médicaux Français (CSMF), older, established physicians, who were less affected by the freeze, squared off against young doctors, especially new specialists, who wished to recoup income they had lost during their long medical training.[23] It had become clear that, if allowed to grow unchecked, the Sector 2 fee waivers would devour the founding promise of *Sécurité Sociale*. As one journalist observed, "If permitted to multiply, medical fee waivers will kill the goose that lays the golden eggs."[24] As in the 1930s and 1950s, doctors' liberty of fees had once again collided head-on with the republic's goal of equality.

Meanwhile, French political leaders' explanations of growing inequalities in U.S. health care fell short. Medical practitioners zealously asserting their liberties were hardly the main cause of care inequities or exorbitant health care inflation in the United States, contrary to what Majnoni d'Intignano had claimed. In fact, in the hands of managed care, U.S. physicians' incomes actually fell in 1993 and 1994, beginning a trend that continued until the end of the century.[25] More important, so many U.S. physicians had come under the sway of managed care's risk/reward incentives that they could hardly be classified as independent political actors in the same sense as their feuding French counterparts. What the two countries did share was a continuing battle with cost control and a growing public malaise about the direction of health care change.

Like the French, Americans were also growing anxious about the two-class health care system. On one side stood those covered by comprehensive private or public health insurance of some kind, for example, Medicare or the Veterans Health Administration. On the other stood Medicaid recipients, the uninsured, and the underinsured. This divide, in and of itself, did not spur reform. The uninsured (mostly the working poor and their children) were too "diffuse, protean, and unorganized" to effectively influence the political debate.[26] Rather, it was the direction of change that precipitated reform efforts. Simply put, more and more Americans feared for their health security. Until 1977, health coverage, whether through private or public insurers, had continued to climb, reaching 87 percent of the population. The 1980s, however, saw a reversal. On the eve of the 1992 presidential contest, the rate of health coverage had fallen to 84 percent of the population; economic recession bred health security fears even among those who enjoyed good coverage.[27] And the loss of one's job (and thereby insurance) through corporate downsizing was not the only threat.

A 1991 court ruling clarified an employer's freedom to drop or modify health benefits under the 1974 Employment Retirement and Income Security Act (ERISA). The case involved John W. McGann who, while working at H & H Music Company, became infected with HIV. As an employee eligible for benefits, McGann sought medical treatment for his condition under the company's insurance, which provided reimbursements of up to 1 million dollars for all diseases. H & H Music Company subsequently changed its health coverage, reducing AIDS-related claims to a lifetime maximum of five thousand dollars. McGann sued under the relevant ERISA section, which prohibits discrimination against an employee "for exercising any right to which he is entitled under the provisions of the employee benefits plan." The Fifth Circuit Court of Appeals, however, adopted the premise that "when an employer's group insurance plan clearly provides that it may be amended or terminated, an employer is free to eliminate the entire plan."[28]

The United States Supreme Court refused to hear the McGann case. But for those who dismissed McGann's plight as having to do more with discrimination against an AIDS patient than with health insurance, the Supreme Court later made its view abundantly clear in a case concerning health benefits for retirees. "Employers or other plan sponsors are generally free under ERISA, for any reason at any time, to adopt, modify, or terminate welfare plans."[29] Hence, workers who believed they were covered through their employers, were, in fact, vulnerable to the company's financial calculations if they required costly care. Indeed, in the case of publicly owned corporations, the rulings could be construed to mean that boards held a fiduciary responsibility to shareholders that trumped ill workers. This was especially true of workers at small firms. There, employers' motivation to change or deny coverage to preserve affordable premiums for the remaining employees was proportionally greater than that of employers at large firms, which could more easily absorb the premium hikes resulting from costly illnesses.

More troubling still, what became known as "the ERISA vacuum" because of the law's prohibition on states regulating employee benefit plans (this power was reserved for the federal government), applied to unions' Taft-Hartley funds and self-insured employers. Through self-insurance, unions and employers saved money by underwriting their own risk pools but usually still hired a health insurer to administer claims and handle relations with medical care providers. The ERISA vacuum prompted an analogous trend among large and even small employers. By 1990, 80 percent of all firms with more than five thousand workers had switched to self-insurance.[30] By 1991, 23 percent of all small employers—that is, those with fewer than a hundred employees—who offered health insurance at all had gone to self-insuring, up from 9 percent only three years earlier.[31]

The prerogative of ERISA-protected health insurance plans to deny coverage brought into question the very definition of insurance. It took the logic of experience rating and permitted insurers and employers to apply it after the fact. As Rand Rosenblatt, a legal scholar of ERISA, testified before a congressional subcommittee, "If insurance companies are justified in 'weeding out' high risk individuals before they gain access to the standard risk pool, does not fairness require that 'standard risk' individuals who gain access to the insured pool *not* be 'weeded out' after their risk has materialized? Is not the whole point of the insurance bargain that a 'standard risk' individual is insured if the (unlikely) risk does occur?"[32] That had certainly been the assumption of most Americans. Nevertheless, the McGann case and those that followed showed otherwise and contributed to a growing unease among supposedly well-covered workers.

The Difficult Art of Reform in the United States

An unusual crystal clear January day in Washington, D.C., lent credence to the buttons proclaiming "A New Beginning" sported by attendees of Bill Clinton's presidential inauguration. But historical developments that had begun in the 1910s shackled the new president's health care reform proposal from its inception: its appeal to the middle class, its preservation of the employment link to health coverage, its respect for private insurers, and its timidity about levying new taxes. This is not to suggest that a different proposal would necessarily have been successful, but rather that the enormous brunt of history and the principles of liberty and equality, always difficult to reconcile, played a key role in the new president's reform effort. Indeed, it was a forthright appeal of health care equality that had attracted the attention of candidate Bill Clinton, but in the end, equality proved to be his proposal's greatest liability.

It began when a little-known political outsider, the Democrat Harris Wofford, who campaigned heavily on the issue of health care insecurity, defeated a heavily favored Republican candidate for a Pennsylvania seat in the United States Senate. Wofford had trailed his rival, Richard Thornburgh, twice elected governor of Pennsylvania, and attorney general in the first Bush administration, by forty-seven points. But Thornburgh's White House ties, a recession, and the dismissive tone he adopted toward his opponent (whom he called "Wooford" when they debated) made him vulnerable. Wofford, a former JFK aide, now president of Bryn Mawr College, replied to Thornburgh's haughtiness with an unabashed demand for health care equality. In his most successful television ad, Wofford stood in a hospital emergency room and boldly stated, "If criminals have a right to a lawyer, I think working Americans should have a right to a doctor.... I'm Harris Wofford, and I believe there is nothing more fundamental than the right to see a doctor when you're sick." [33] After Wofford's upset victory, polls showed that 71 percent of his voters reported health care as either the first or second most important reason for their vote. Clinton took note and hired Wofford's chief political consultants. [34]

In a way, Clinton represented the ideal reformer because he held no hard-and-fast convictions about how to change U.S. health care. He nevertheless grasped what mattered most: the need to rescue and revamp a beleaguered system in order to improve efficiency and expand coverage. [35] He was certainly no revolutionary. In these traits, Clinton shared much with the twentieth century's most successful reformers. As the historian Robert Skidelsky deftly puts it, "Social systems are never saved by true believers, the virtues appropriate to going down with the ship rarely being suitable to the arts of navigation." [36]

Even before his inauguration, Clinton faced fateful decisions in the treacherous waters of health care reform. The choices and their variants were many, yet they generally fell into three camps: 1) expand Medicare into a single payer for all, effectively building on the Roosevelt administration's original plan to include health security as part of Social Security; 2) mandate that employers either provide health insurance or pay a substitute tax to cover workers by other means, also known as "play or pay"; 3) introduce market-oriented voluntary measures, such as tax incentives and small business insurance-purchasing groups, which could stabilize and expand coverage. Because defeated president George H. W. Bush had centered his own health care campaign around option three (which candidate Clinton had duly attacked), this left only two possible options for the new occupant of the White House.

History weighed heavily on both. Despite its intuitive simplicity and the Congressional Budget Office's judgment as to its cost-effectiveness, the single-payer option never received serious consideration. First, as an expansion of Medicare's contributory social insurance approach, it would have meant a massive reorientation of funds away from private insurers and toward some sort of public agency, which in turn would have paid medical care providers or contracted with insurers (now skeletons of their former selves) to administer the program. Powerful health insurance lobbies would have fought a single-payer proposal to the death, a battle the new president apparently saw as futile.

Second, many of the most powerful unions remained committed to employment-based health care. After all, their members had largely gained health coverage at the collective bargaining table or through their use of Taft-Hartley funds, both of which relied on experience-rated insurance to keep their comprehensive benefits affordable. To be sure, labor leaders had maintained a steady drumbeat for health care reform, which sometimes included advocacy of a single-payer system, and they, like employers, railed against health care inflation. Yet when change appeared likely in the early 1990s, AFL-CIO president Lane Kirkland teamed with John J. Sweeney, leader of the influential Service Employees International Union, to block the influence of those who advocated a single-payer option.[37]

Third, Clinton, as a self-described "new Democrat," wanted little to do with the New Deal and Great Society programs of the Roosevelt and Johnson eras. He had, in fact, run against "big government" and had insisted from the beginning that his reform would entail no new taxes. If he proposed a single-payer reform, critics could have tagged him a hypocrite and, if U.S. history is any guide, a Communist in disguise who wanted to "socialize" U.S. medicine.[38] By the same logic, Clinton officials avoided any mention of foreign models, including the Canadian, or even France's more balanced public-private health care system.

This left "play or pay," but that option by itself failed to deal with the other imperative of health care reform: cost control. Here Clinton was forced to improvise. He proposed the creation of regional health alliances, quasi-governmental organizations through which employers, even small ones, could purchase community-rated insurance at competitive prices. In competition to sell their policies to the health alliances, insurers would themselves control prices through the use of managed care, which by the early 1990s was spreading quickly in U.S. medicine. Thus, next to "managed care," the Clinton plan added "managed competition" to the lexicon of health care reform. To the dismay of some health insurers, however, Clinton also proposed "backstop" premium caps, which could have been activated in the event prices rose too quickly. But because organizations that exceeded five thousand workers could opt out of health alliance participation, his plan permitted maximum maneuvering room for large employers and the unions' Taft-Hartley funds.

If the Clinton Health Care Task Force, led by First Lady Hillary Rodham Clinton, successfully navigated the most treacherous obstacles to health care reform, they failed to engender a broad positive consensus. True, they avoided a frontal attack on insurers, widespread higher taxes, and new restrictions on physician liberties or patient choice, and they made plausible promises to improve many Americans' health coverage and security. Indeed, the basic benefit package compared favorably with comprehensive benefits offered by the country's largest corporations.[39] Yet like the American Association of Labor Legislation (AALL) in 1916, which had attempted to enact compulsory health insurance, the Clinton administration failed to elicit sufficient grassroots support for its plan. This permitted opponents to transform indifferent observers into an effective coalition of the fearful. At root lay the president's relations with unions, which was yet another characteristic that Clinton shared with the AALL of 1916.

It appeared that unions had much to gain from Clinton's centrist reform proposal and that labor leaders would be able to rally massive support to assure its legislative victory in a Democrat-controlled Congress. This calculation, however, ignored a nearly simultaneous battle over the North American Free Trade Agreement (NAFTA) in the fall of 1993, which the president supported and unions vociferously opposed. Threatened with the loss of additional well-paid manufacturing jobs to Mexico, labor leaders forged a formidable coalition with environmental, farm, consumer, and civil rights groups to block NAFTA. In response, Clinton launched his own all-out campaign of presidential arm-twisting and promise making on Capitol Hill. When the votes were counted in the House of Representatives, the president prevailed, but only by relying on thirty more votes from Republicans than from his fellow Democrats. Having "kicked sand in labor's face," Clinton then appealed for their help to pass health care reform.[40] Even an otherwise optimistic internal White House memo conceded that the NAFTA fight had left a "residue of anger and bitterness" from which it would take AFL-CIO unions "a while to cool off."[41] But "a while" was exactly what the administration did not have.

A lull in labor and associated public interest group support for the president gave Clinton's opponents valuable time. They effectively played on the complexity of his proposal—all 1,342 pages of it. Perhaps the most successful attack came from the Health Insurance Association of America with its "Harry and Louise" television spots. Harry and Louise, a middle-aged couple who enjoy insurance but nonetheless profess support for reform, sit at their kitchen table and grow confused and fearful about what Clinton's regional health care alliances would mean for them. The "Harry and Louise" spots represented a "we've got ours" counterpoint to Harris Wofford's television spot in the hospital emergency room demanding health care equality. The security of Harry and Louise's kitchen provides a marked contrast to the insecurity—physical and financial—of Wofford's ER. If Wofford focused on the falling rate of employment-based insurance, "Harry and Louise" targeted the 54.2 percent of Americans who, in 1992, still enjoyed health care security through employment-based coverage (even though that number had fallen from 61.2 percent in 1979).[42]

Compared with previous health care reform battles, the fight over the Clinton plan caused relatively little divisiveness among physicians. In part this was because the principal battles over medical practice freedoms lay in the private sector, between doctors and managed care insurers. This being the case, medical leaders wanted first and foremost to channel reform so that it protected fee-for-service practices and patient choice. Toward this end, medical leaders variously supported either employer mandates or, as in the case of the American College of Surgeons, the expansion of Medicare.[43] For their part, AMA leaders wanted to require employers to provide coverage of their full-time workers and foresaw an expanded Medicaid program that covered part-timers. This they championed under the banner "Health Access America." But AMA leaders were clearly disposed to compromise with the president on the basis of "play or pay."

The editor of the *Journal of the American Medical Association,* George Lundberg, opined in May 1993 that Hawaii's employer mandate law—the only one in the nation—was a "beautiful blend of civilized cooperation, coverage, and professionalism.... Making it national, almost as is, would be a huge improvement over what we have."[44] For this and other non-specific but supportive gestures toward the Clinton plan, the AMA itself became the object of a lobbying campaign by the National Federation of Independent Businesses, whose members, mostly small business owners, opposed employer mandates. Magnifying their influence, the Republican national leadership took up the cause of small businesses. Future House Speaker Newt Gingrich drafted a letter to all 450 members of the AMA's House of Delegates, chastising the AMA for being "out of touch with rank and file physicians."[45]

In her account of the politics surrounding the Clinton initiative, the sociologist Theda Skocpol demonstrates the extent to which Republican leaders such as Gingrich effectively harnessed confusion and misgivings about the Clinton plan and transformed them into a broad attack on New Deal and Great Society social programs, an attack begun under Ronald Reagan.[46] But if astute politics reinvigorated Republicans' offensive against the welfare state, the raw material for Clinton's failure lay in the United States' historical embrace of private voluntary health insurance and employment-based coverage. As the political scientist Marie Gottschalk explains, "These institutions helped realign the interests of labor more closely with those of business and the insurers. They also contributed to tensions within and among unions and liberal-leaning public-interest groups... [and] made it that much more difficult for labor to lead rather than follow in the health-care reform debate."[47]

Ultimately, in the absence of broad and enthusiastic grassroots support, which labor failed to provide, opponents of the Clinton plan successfully counterpoised those who had health coverage against those who did not. By the close of 1994, the Clinton plan had become lost in a sea of competing congressional proposals and deliberations, and never reached the floor of either house for a vote.

The Difficult Art of Reform in France

Bill Clinton's debacle attracted considerable attention in France, not least because, as in the United States of 1992, some sort of health care reform was widely viewed as inevitable. The issue remained how best to go about it. In September 1995, *Le Monde* ran a front-page editorial on exactly this question. The paper contrasted Germany's success at enacting health care reform with the United States' failure. "The 'German method' has been shown far more efficient," observed *Le Monde*. "It led to real negotiations among responsible societal actors...and has been signed by the federal government, the states, employers, workers' unions, the medical professions, and beneficiaries." In contrast, the article continued, "The 'Clinton method' has been a calamity.... Aided by a vast cohort of 'experts'... [it] created a gigantic document that would have radically reorganized, to the smallest detail, the American health care system.... [The] pseudo-negotiations over interests...allowed lobbies time...to attack the proposal. Fearful for their 'acquired rights,' they blocked reform."[48] The erroneous characterization of Clinton's proposal as a radical reorganization of U.S. health care aside, *Le Monde* correctly captured basic differences between how Germans and Americans approach social reform.

Social scientists often explain the distinction between the politics of the United States and those of European parliamentary democracies by relying on what they call "peak associations." A peak association is a corporatist institution that can authoritatively speak with a single voice for a broad set of interest groups.[49] Certainly, the existence of powerful and popularly supported peak associations to represent German workers, employers, and physicians proved critical to the success of Germany's 1994 health care reforms. *Le Monde* was contrasting the U.S. and German cases in order to advocate what is known in France as *concertation*, a process by which authoritative representatives of all stakeholders negotiate simultaneously with government officials and with one another to reach an accord.

By contrast, the Clinton Health Care Task Force, which *Le Monde* dismissed as a "cohort of 'experts,'" preferred one-on-one meetings with health care lobbies and actors, which bred suspicion and led some to throw in their lot with congressional opponents and others to take to the airwaves in efforts to get a better deal from the administration.[50] But though France possessed a more unified governmental structure than the United States, which made *concertation* a plausible option, it lacked German-style peak associations. Indeed, French health care politics, with their competing medical *syndicats*, rival workers' unions, and disparate employer interests, resemble U.S. pluralism far more than German corporatism.[51] In fact, the sharp divisions within and among various stakeholders led the government of Prime Minister Edouard Balladur in 1994 to create a commission of experts on health care. Their charge was to examine "the deep crisis" of French health care, which, "beyond the current economic recession...is the result of an insufficient control of expenditures."[52] Their report, Balladur hoped, would provide a road map of reform options to the nation's leaders.

Yet rather than a considered exploration of options, the commission's report reads more like a map of a historical legacy, telling leaders where they could *not* go. The most forbidden lands were those that restricted customary liberties. The authors insist that "private-practice medicine rests on an ancient tradition to which patients and medical professionals alike are legitimately attached. To challenge it would be both futile and dangerous." Readers are likewise urged to avoid venturing toward a "two-class health care system." They must remember that "inequality before sickness is among the most despicable circumstances. . . . This would be the case if the poorest had access to but one sort of care."[53] Above all, revolutionary action was explicitly prohibited. Just as history warned the Clinton team away from serious consideration of a single-payer option, the commission report urged French leaders to "mistrust entirely new systems that are presented as total solutions and which often take their inspiration from how things are done elsewhere. . . . To be a fundamentalist in reform leads to inaction."[54]

Although a makeover of French health care was ruled out as unrealistic, the authors appeared more sanguine about an even more unlikely event: the voluntary transformation of doctors and patients into self-rationing providers and consumers of medical care. Physicians were simply urged to become more "virtuous." They should "cut down on unjustified therapies and prescriptions . . . and accept alternative modes of remuneration such as capitated payments instead of a fee for each service." Patients were likewise encouraged to "renounce direct access to specialists, except in special cases . . . abandon seeking several medical opinions . . . practice prevention . . . [and] find a virtuous doctor."[55] The expert authors of the report had scant advice about how political leaders should enforce virtue. But this did not prevent a newly elected prime minister from trying.

In France's semipresidential system, the president must work in tandem with a prime minister in domestic affairs. The prime minister is conventionally drawn from the National Assembly's dominant party. Jacques Chirac's victory in the 1995 presidential contest also brought to power his own coalition of center-right parties in the Assembly, which permitted Chirac to select a trusted protégé, Alain Juppé, as prime minister. Chirac urged a seemingly impossible balance between consensus building and action. "One must act quickly but also give reform a chance. There's a time for *concertation*, which has to be sufficient. There's a time for a decision and for implementation, which has to be short."[56]

Trying to act on Chirac's advice, Juppé moved quickly to prepare a sweeping plan, but, like Clinton, he soon lost momentum in the face of fierce opposition. Less than six months after taking office, Juppé unveiled *Sécurité Sociale* reforms that he claimed had been "guided by three ideas: exigency, justice, and responsibility." He staked his claim to exigency on growing *Sécurité Sociale* deficits, which previous reforms had attempted to solve by relying on increased payroll and other taxes. By 1994, employer and employee contributions, which remained the predominant form of health insurance funding, had reached 19.6 percent of gross wages. Of that employers paid 12.8 percent and employees contributed 6.8 percent. "Everyone agrees," Juppé surmised, "that the present financing is unfavorable to employment because taxes on wages make the cost of labor so expensive."[57] Hence, Juppé proposed a partial abandonment of employment-based financing of *Sécurité Sociale* by increasing its reliance on an income tax, the Contribution Sociale Généralisée (CSG). This, it was hoped, would dampen the country's corrosive unemployment rate, which had hovered at around 10 percent since the 1980s. If only employers did not face such high nonwage labor costs, Juppé believed, they would hire more workers. Higher employment, in turn, would translate into greater personal income (and lower unemployment insurance payouts), which would, of course, bring more revenue to *Sécurité Sociale*.

A shift away from payroll levies toward the new CSG income tax also contributed to Juppé's vision of a more just *Sécurité Sociale*. As early as the 1940s, the founding director of *Sécurité Sociale*, Pierre Laroque, had questioned the fairness of requiring workers alone to pay for an increasingly generous welfare state that benefited much of the population.[58] By 1995 the problem had become much worse. True, 99 percent of France's population enjoyed health care coverage and virtually all of them were subject to *Sécurité Sociale* wage taxes to pay for it. But that still left whole classes of income earners, those whose revenue came from rents and investments, for example, who made relatively small sacrifices to enjoy one of the most generous and technologically advanced health care systems in the world.

Juppé's plan to increase the CSG's bite on unearned income represented an important divergence in France's health care financing away from a structural feature it had long shared with its U.S. counterpart. Perhaps even more so than Americans, the French have long been hostile to income taxes, and their governments have relied on them only sparingly.

At the time of Juppé's proposal, only half of all households were subject to income taxes and even then the tax was levied on only half of their income. Popular dislike of income taxes was reinforced by a historical acceptance of wage levies, an acceptance on which *Sécurité Sociale* had been built. This, as much as anything, explains why Juppé could propose only a limited replacement of wage levies with income taxes.[59]

Even after Juppé's reform, French workers still paid for 75 percent of their health care through insurance premiums deducted from their paychecks.[60] *Sécurité Sociale* thereby preserved the link between worker and beneficiary, which had deep historical roots in the mutual movement of the nineteenth century and interwar years. France could not, after all, transform itself overnight into a Scandinavian country such as Denmark, where local property and income taxes paid for 80 percent of its public health care system.[61] Employers and labor leaders alike understood that if health insurance premiums were "fiscalized," that is, transferred to a generalized income tax, their claims to control *Sécurité Sociale* governing boards would surely diminish. This was a prospect to which they were determinedly opposed.[62] Finally, in the same way that U.S. firms and workers had grown accustomed to the tax deductibility of their health insurance premiums, French workers had come to enjoy the tax-exempt status of their employer-provided supplemental health insurance, which presented yet another obstacle to Juppé's reform plan.

Supplemental health insurance coverage had become all the more important after 1970 as reformers attempted to "take advantage of market forces" by permitting physicians more fee-setting liberties and by passing more costs on to patients. Between 1980 and 1987, reimbursements for all medical care slipped about a half a percent per year. By 1994, at an average of 59.5 percent, France possessed the lowest reimbursement rate for ambulatory care among the fifteen countries of the European Union (EU). France also accounted for 20 percent of the EU's private health insurance reimbursements and out-of-pocket medical expenses. As a result, fully 83 percent of the population had obtained supplemental health coverage, either from a growing private, for-profit insurance industry—in 1995 estimated at 25 percent of the market—or from the country's traditional nonprofit mutual societies. Half of all supplemental coverage was provided through the workplace.[63]

Even though *Sécurité Sociale* remained foundational to France's health care system, private supplemental health insurance had grown so widespread that it prevented Juppé from seeking a massive change in how workers obtained health coverage, just as the long attachment to employment-based private health insurance in the United States blocked reform there. If Alain Juppé had proposed Danish-style income taxes to pay for health care, it would have been akin to Bill Clinton announcing his intention to adopt a Canadian-style single-payer plan. For historical reasons, neither leader deemed these choices politically viable, at least not in the mid-1990s. Sadly, both nations' long history of contributory workplace health coverage proved too heavy a burden on otherwise able reformers.

Whether in the case of early French mutual societies, U.S. Blue Cross hospital plans, or later employment-based health insurance (*Sécurité Sociale* or Blue Shield), the concept, "I work, therefore I'm covered," took root during the formative stages of health security in both countries. The link between employment and health security thus came to underlie the notion of "deserving" and "less deserving" citizens. In the United States, both Medicare and employment-based private health insurance created an ethos according to which only those who had contributed at the workplace had rights, even if these programs also relied heavily on general tax revenues (Medicare) or tax subsidies (employment-based insurance). Medicaid, meanwhile, a far less generous program for the working poor and indigent who lacked access to affordable employment-based coverage, quite explicitly took the place of physicians' charity, but charity it remained. Compared with Medicare, Medicaid entails few rights and fewer political supporters.

Albeit less pronounced, France's comparable historical tradition of workplace health coverage underlies inequities of health care access because of the continued importance of supplemental insurance. Although 83 percent of the population had obtained private supplemental coverage by 1995, these benefits were not equitably distributed across socioeconomic lines. Only 68 percent of skilled wage earners enjoyed supplemental insurance, compared with 90 percent of white-collar managers.[64] What is more, a recent study that controlled for socioeconomic and demographic factors and health status found that French adults with supplemental insurance are 86 percent more likely to seek medical care than those without such coverage. This disparity nearly matches that found between the likelihood of insured and uninsured adult Americans seeking care, even though the financial burden of treatment for uninsured Americans is far greater than that of those who lack supplemental coverage in France.[65]

If Alain Juppé could not entirely break his countrymen's and -women's attachment to workplace health insurance—despite its inequities—he was determined to achieve universal coverage. This he accomplished under the heading of "justice." Ever so carefully, Juppé announced: "We will create, first of all, a universal system of health insurance.... This will not mean a 'single system' [for everybody]; it will remain compatible with employment-based [health insurance] funds."[66] The Couverture Médicale Universelle (CMU) was hardly shocking. It steered well clear of a major reorganization of existing insurance funds by merely simplifying enrollment and rationalizing needlessly complex relations between *Sécurité Sociale* funds and those of certain sectors, such as the national railroad and metro transit, whose health insurance funds remained technically outside *Sécurité Sociale*.[67]

The CMU assured *Sécurité Sociale* and a modicum of supplemental insurance coverage for those who were between jobs, the indigent, and others who had somehow fallen through the cracks. Certainly, the CMU marked an important milestone in France's health care system. But it was far from a major structural change. Like the limited transformation of some wage levies into income taxes, the achievement of universal coverage evoked little surprise or controversy. Neither measure threatened powerful lobbies or well-organized beneficiaries. Things were decidedly different, however, for changes that Juppé proposed under the heading of "responsibility."

For Juppé, responsibility meant, above all, the financial sustainability of the health care system. He proposed that Parliament and *Sécurité Sociale* boards, "in consultation with an annual health conference, [set] spending rates by sector" in order to create a national health care budget. What was more, a revamped process that reduced the power of unions relative to employers would modify the selection of *Sécurité Sociale* board members. As if unions were not a formidable enough opponent, Juppé fleshed out his proposal to control health care costs with special attention to physicians. "We will put in place automatic adjustments to doctors' pay that correspond to [their] respect of [spending] goals; specifically, this will mean that fee increases will from now on be conditional and temporary."

Furthermore, new restrictions on physicians' clinical freedoms were to be governed by an accelerated "development of 'best medical practices'" that would weed out extravagant therapies and unnecessary prescriptions based on professional and scientific norms.[68] Physicians had earlier agreed to such a *maîtrise médicalisée* of cost, a term they preferred because it emphasized the medico-scientific as opposed to the financial-political modes of stemming utilization. They had also accepted a limited list of pathologies, determined by the new medical reference guides. Yet, from the physicians' point of view, Juppé's reform plan would involve a vast expansion of the program without sufficient consultation.[69]

Nor did patient liberties escape unscathed. Taking a page from the U.S. managed care handbook, Juppé proposed "experimentation with new forms of care, namely, the requirement to see a general practitioner before going to a specialist." Also, to prevent patients from seeking redundant care and multiple pharmaceutical prescriptions for the same condition, all consulted physicians would have access to a digitized medical chart for each patient.[70] As one observer noted, with only slight exaggeration, "France is the only country in the world where one could get eighteen electrocardiograms in nine days—one in the morning, one in the evening, and be reimbursed without a single question asked."[71] The necessary funds for the information technology to computerize patient charts were to be raised by a small tax on every reimbursement form submitted to *Sécurité Sociale*.

If the sheer scope of his plan to enforce "responsibility" in health care utilization was not provocative enough, Juppé broke a cardinal rule that had long been observed by would-be government health care reformers on both sides of the Atlantic. He mentioned the word *rationing*, albeit to deny its existence. "We refuse," insisted Juppé, "to even consider the path of health care rationing or the reduction of [patient] reimbursements."[72] In response, Claude Maffioli, the president of France's largest physician's association, the CSMF, made sure that in the weeks following the announcement of Juppé's plan, the public heard the word "rationing" as often as possible. Maffioli added other liberty-offending terms to elicit the maximum negative emotional response from the public, most of whom had long enjoyed vast freedoms of patient choice and virtually unlimited access to medical services. "They're imposing a bookkeeping cost control guided by a mandatory rate fixed unilaterally without any consideration of real needs. It's the path of rationing."[73] Three days later, Maffioli added: "Are the French really ready to put their names on waiting lists for surgery as in Great Britain?"[74] Doctors, Maffioli announced, would educate patients in their offices through posters and handouts regarding the dangers of Juppé's plan for health care. With the exception of the general practitioners' association, MG-France, whose leadership supported the notion of gatekeeping primary care physicians, all the country's medical leaders lined up to oppose the Juppé plan. Not surprisingly, the dreaded label "health care rationing" stuck. And for good reason. Parliament proposed limiting 1996 increases for ambulatory care to 2.1 percent, well below the 1995 target rate of 3.3 percent, and far under the actual 1995 increase of 6.7 percent.[75]

With doctors emphasizing the specter of "health care rationing," Minister of Labor and Social Affairs Jacques Barrot fought back with a rhetorical offensive of his own. "Don't you think we're going to get around the lobbies!" he responded to a skeptical journalist.[76] By using the English word "lobby," which in France connotes a purely financially motivated interest group, Barrot hoped to deny doctors their preferred public persona as protectors of health care quality and patients. But the offensive fell flat. Unions, including the dominant CGT and the FO, had already launched street protests against rises in public sector workers' retirement age, another key provision of the Juppé plan that addressed *Sécurité Sociale* pension deficits. By mid-December, the street marches had mushroomed into the largest strikes and demonstrations that France had seen since the massive social unrest of May 1968. Despite their sometime testy relations with labor leaders, doctors benefited from the widespread public support for unions in their battle against pension reforms. Unions' success at painting Juppé as an extremist bent on dismantling *Sécurité Sociale,* on its fiftieth anniversary no less, proved too much for the government to withstand.

In early January, after a two-hour meeting with medical leaders, and just two months after announcing his plan, Juppé withdrew major aspects of his proposal. Physician fees would not be withheld by *Sécurité Sociale* to enforce expanded clinical practice norms. And the tax on patient reimbursement forms, which would have been spent on computerizing doctors' medical records, was formally withdrawn. With neither sanctions to delimit extraordinary therapeutic practices nor any way to track patients who sought redundant care, Juppé had been forced to abandon the principal levers of health care cost control.[77] Further rationalization of hospital spending and a limited transfer of wage levies to the CSG income tax survived the public outpouring of discontent. In due course, Parliament also adopted annual national health care spending objectives as called for in the Juppé plan, but government and *Sécurité Sociale* leaders still lacked sufficient means to enforce them. Indeed, France's "global health care budget," which was supposed to bring health care inflation in line with economic growth and general price rises, has been surpassed virtually every year since its approval.[78]

Many general practitioners supported the Juppé plan or at least held their fire, an indication of a critical change under way within the medical profession. Although still far from the U.S. model, under which roughly two-thirds of medical students become specialists, the French medical profession saw more and more French doctors staying in school for specialty training. Indeed, by 1995 the growth in primary care physicians had come to a standstill, while the number of specialists had continued to grow at an annual average rate of 4.8 percent since 1987, making up 44 percent of the profession by 1996.[79]

The shifting balance between specialists and primary care physicians has coincided with France's growing reliance on supplemental health insurance. Specialists were far more likely to set up practice as Sector 2 physicians, thereby escaping adherence to standard *Sécurité Sociale* fees to which Sector 1 doctors were bound. Under these conditions, more specialists have inevitably meant higher patient bills, which *Sécurité Sociale* reimbursed at lower rates. This progression, in turn, helped drive the expansion of France's private insurance industry in the 1980s and 1990s. For only through supplemental coverage could patients escape paying the higher fees entirely out of their own pockets. The greater proportion of specialists also helped undercut the influence of Juppé's call for gatekeeping doctors and his hopes to reorient and rationalize patient care through them. Even before Juppé had launched his reform effort, a former director of the *Sécurité Sociale* health insurance fund, Gilles Johanet, warned, "France is progressively leaving the European model behind and is becoming American."[80]

Reflections on the Difficult Art of Health Care Reform

When all was said and done, the Clinton and Juppé reforms were caught in a three-way collision between health care inflation, historically entrenched health care interests, and a public with an idealized conception of medical care. In both nations, employers, physicians, insurers, and unions, though far from reading from a common script, acted or failed to act to stymie reform. Mistrust of "the system," which grew out of the social unrest of the 1960s and 1970s, combined with an economic downturn and the medical care cost explosion to sap public support for health care change. Without a sufficiently positive consensus, or what the French term *concertation*, the Clinton and Juppé plans became sitting ducks for interest groups that might otherwise have been forced to compromise.

Unions occupied a critical position in both nations. In both cases, they tipped the balance against reform, in part because of coincident events but also because of unions' historical privileges. Juppé's larger plan included pension reform, which gave rise to fierce opposition among public sector workers, the most unionized portion of France's otherwise scantily organized labor force. Hundreds of thousands took to the streets against *le plan Juppé*, signaling opposition to the entirety of reform and its vulgar representation as the dismantling of *Sécurité Sociale*. Under these circumstances, with their health care access and choice intact, workers had little incentive to acquiesce to complex health care changes that might muddy their struggle against pension reform.

Juppé's pension reform was to France what Clinton's dogged pursuit of NAFTA was to the United States. It poisoned a well of potential support for health care change. Into each circumstance stepped irreversibly opposed interest groups—doctors in the case of France and insurers and small businesses in the case of the United States. Their campaigns against reform gained handsomely from the divided attitudes of labor. If U.S. workers with good health insurance did not take to the streets like their French counterparts, they hardly mobilized in favor of the Clinton plan either. More likely, they were at home, watching the Health Insurance Association of America's "Harry and Louise" spots, which questioned why anyone with good health coverage would risk a change.

In the aftermath of the Juppé and Clinton reform efforts, pieces of their initiatives were approved. Juppé's plans for new funding sources and a rationalization of the hospital sector gained approval in 1996. His successor in the prime minister's office, the Socialist Lionel Jospin, enacted the Couverture Médicale Universelle, which ensured health coverage to all citizens and permanent residents by 2000. Juppé's vision of ambulatory "health care pathways" headed by gatekeeping primary care physicians also became reality in late 1997, albeit on a voluntary basis (for patient and doctor), and only because the government offered financial incentives to both. Thus, even though massive strikes and demonstrations against Alain Juppé's larger Sécurité Sociale proposals forced his resignation, his health care initiatives marked the beginning of fruitful reform.

The same cannot be said of Bill Clinton's plan. Its utter failure effectively ruled out any major health care reform attempts for nearly ten years. True, congressional backers of the Clinton Health Care plan succeeded in passing legislation that improved insurance coverage for children of poor households and provided a modicum of health security for some who were between jobs, the Health Insurance Portability and Accountability Act of 1996. But in contrast to the French legislation that followed Juppé's departure, neither measure had been central to Clinton's larger reform plan. Clinton could not claim, as Juppé ultimately could, that his defeat had not been in vain, that he had, in fact, pushed forward durable and productive health care reform even if much remained to be done.

More so than in France, U.S. health care change since the defeat of the Clinton plan demonstrates the extent to which historically powerful actors hold sway. The Medicare Modernization Act of 2003, which created a much-needed prescription drug benefit for the elderly, further empowers a labyrinth of powerful health insurers and pharmaceutical companies that provide some (but by no means all) Americans with health security. Some seniors may be better off because of the new law, but a historic opportunity was missed to make more sweeping Medicare reforms that would ensure its long-term viability.

A 2004 General Accounting Office report predicts that Medicare expenditures will grow by 99 percent in real dollars by 2013, fueled by retiring baby boomers and continued steep health care inflation.[81] The Medicare reform of 2003 fails to grapple with such a scenario. Instead, private insurers gained new financial incentives to practice their well-honed skills of risk selection, thereby competing to enroll healthier than average seniors at least as much as they provide quality services to beneficiaries. To wit, after passage of the reform, Florida retirement communities that cater to golf-playing seniors enjoyed daily free lunches from five different health insurers seeking to have them enroll in Medicare managed care plans. It is doubtful that these insurers extended the same largesse to skilled nursing facilities in hopes of enrolling chronically ill Medicare patients whose medical care utilization per beneficiary is much higher. Indeed, data submitted by the private managed care plans themselves indicate that they serve beneficiaries for whom expected costs were 8 percent lower than the typical fee-for-service Medicare beneficiary. Meanwhile, the Medicare Modernization Act of 2003 pays them 108 percent of what it pays for a traditional Medicare beneficiary, a projected 46 billion dollars over the next ten years. And government officials expect a tripling of Medicare managed care enrollees, to one in three of all beneficiaries, as the new Medicare legislation comes into force.[82]

As with the disparity between mid-century health coverage for unionized industrial workers and nonunion agricultural laborers, risk selection through experience-rated insurance leads to vast racial, class, and gender inequalities in health care security. Some seniors will no doubt benefit from lower co-payments in managed care plans, just as they do from the new prescription drug rules, but the structural fragmentation of the Medicare risk pool (at public expense no less) is not sustainable in light of continued health care inflation and demographic change. Elements of managed care may well be part of the solution to Medicare's challenges. But the 2003 reform hearkens back to the 1950s, when the Eisenhower administration encouraged the spread of private voluntary insurance through generous government subsidies, namely, the tax deductibility of group health insurance premiums. We can now see that this path ultimately proved very expensive (in forgone tax revenue) and relatively inefficient in bringing about widespread coverage.

Another provision of the 2003 Medicare Modernization Act attempts to stem rising health insurance premiums through what are known as "health savings accounts" (HSAs). Here again, the initiative recalls past eras when both France and the United States attempted to "take advantage of the market" to solve mounting health care crises. An individual who opens an HSA may receive and carry over funds for routine medical care from year to year, but that carryover must be coupled with a high deductible health insurance policy ($1,050 for individuals or $2,100 for families in 2006). By law, an HSA holder cannot also enjoy more comprehensive health coverage. One purpose of HSAs is to make patients more cost-conscious about routine, noncatastrophic medical care. Proponents argue that patients who must pay with what is transparently their own money (out of their HSA) will curb unnecessary care, thereby helping to dampen demand-driven health care inflation.[83] As President George W. Bush explained, "When you go to buy a car, you know, you're able to shop and compare."[84]

A similar reasoning drove Prime Minister Raymond Barre's initiative, which created Sector 2 medical practices in the 1980s. Physicians who declared their practices under Sector 2 could essentially ignore standard fee schedules; they instead had to prove the worth of their more expensive services to consumers in the marketplace. Yet the French quickly learned that the selection of a medical care provider depends as much on a patient's geographic location, her financial means, and her knowledge of her condition as it does on price. As many specialists declared their practices under Sector 2, patients who needed care within a reasonable distance from their home had no choice but to either pay higher fees out of pocket or to not seek care. For them, there were no market choices.

Health savings accounts present a similar problem for Americans who possess neither sufficient means of transportation nor savings to take advantage of a medical marketplace. One study predicts that 44 percent of those with incomes below thirty-five thousand dollars and deductibles higher than five hundred dollars will face significant cost-related access problems with HSAs. The rate for higher-income, insured adults with more traditional coverage is 21 percent.[85] As the French found out by the early 1990s, unleashing market forces in health care, even for routine or preventive ambulatory services, is highly problematic. Time and again over the last century, health care has shown itself resistant to solutions that rely on market forces alone.[86] Nor are health savings accounts expected to make much of a difference in lowering the number of uninsured. Indeed, the health economist Jonathan Gruber believes that HSAs could actually raise the number of uninsured Americans because only about half of workers who are dropped by employer coverage enroll elsewhere.[87]

Even though Alain Juppé's reform plan ultimately resulted in more health care gains by century's end, neither France nor the United States has overcome the main challenge that had moved to the fore after 1970: to slow health care inflation, which is vital to the long-term sustainability of their respective health care systems. What is worse is that U.S. leaders have grown embarrassingly remiss in providing reliable and affordable health security to growing sectors of the U.S. population.

9

LES JEUX SONT FAITS?
2000–PRESENT

Man is condemned to be free; because once thrown into the world, he is responsible for everything he does.

JEAN-PAUL SARTRE, *Existentialism and Human Emotion*

In 1943 the French writer Jean-Paul Sartre published a play entitled *Les Jeux Sont Faits* (*The Chips Are Down*). Set in an unnamed city bringing to mind France under German occupation during the Second World War, it is a story about our inability to be free of our pasts. The main characters, Eve and Pierre, meet in the afterlife, only to discover that a terrible mistake has been made. Both have just been murdered by trusted friends; she by her husband, he by a fellow insurgent. But according to a distressed heavenly official, they were supposed to have met, fallen in love, and become lifelong soul mates. Unwilling to accept this violation of destiny, heavenly authorities insist that Eve and Pierre be given a second chance. They are promptly returned to the living and permitted to escape their respective murderers for twenty-four hours. In order to truly get back their lives beyond the one-day reprieve, they must fulfill their future by falling in love. Yet for all their efforts, Eve and Pierre fail at this life-or-death imperative. What prevents them is not their incompatibility. They are, indeed, meant to be lovers. It is their pasts. Eve and Pierre could not return to their respective lives without getting caught up in the rivalries that resulted in their deaths, ultimately twice over.

Like so many of Sartre's works, *Les Jeux Sont Faits* makes us reflect on what we mean by individual "liberty" in an absurd world. If read as a social allegory, it reminds us of the notion of "path dependency," according to which political-institutional developments are subject to an imperious momentum, pushed down a path whose direction is more likely to be reinforced than abandoned at each juncture. From more or less common beginnings early in the century, historically unique circumstances have led to a wide divergence in French and U.S. health care. Diverse conditions and events exerted formative influences, which in turn led to others, which now make radical reversals difficult. Yet in so many ways, French and U.S. health care, like Eve and Pierre, remain soul mates: not because of any preordained destiny but rather because of the eighteenth-century revolutions that enshrined liberty beside equality, and because of their common struggles, past and present, which stem from these Enlightenment ideals. Eve and Pierre met tragic fates because of their inability to recognize and act on their own liberty. What lies in store for the Americans and the French in pursuit of health?

Will we remain enslaved by our twentieth-century pasts? Before the Americans and the French can even begin to tackle the current problems, we must accurately conceptualize the challenges before us. Comparative history helps us do that, for it lays bare the contours of the past relative to "another" past, drawing more clearly than national histories alone the cultural and material underpinnings of cause and effect. When these causes and effects are illuminated by a century-long comparative history of health care, it becomes apparent that citizens in both the United States and France suffer from troublesome misconceptions about the historical underpinnings of their health care systems and powerfully entrenched interests, both of which will hamper productive national debates over current dilemmas.

Americans remain vexed over whether the country should "go public" or keep its "private" health care system. Do we want "socialized medicine," like the Europeans have, or should we "let the market" provide our health care needs? In 1918, or even as late as 1947, these questions still made some sense. But today they are false dichotomies that cloud Americans' thinking; they stand in the way of an honest reckoning with the past, which is our only way forward.

U.S. health care, like French health care, is a mixed public-private endeavor. Indeed, one of the most obvious trends of the last century is health care's increasing reliance on public financing. In this, the United States differs from France only in degree. Americans have been socializing more and more of the cost of their health care expenses since the Internal Revenue Service ruled in the 1930s that group insurance premiums were tax deductible; legislation codified that rule in 1954. These developments both shaped and spurred the spread of workplace health security. The creation of Medicare and Medicaid in 1965, the swelling list of their beneficiaries since then, and Medicare's expansion in 2003 also mark milestones in the socialization of U.S. medicine. A review of the party affiliation of U.S. presidents and of congressional majorities reveals that these developments cannot be tagged as either Republican or Democratic.

They are part and parcel of deeper social and demographic trends that transcend the relatively narrow (compared with France) U.S. political spectrum. For all the self-perceived exceptionalism on both sides of the Atlantic, the growing role of medical insurance and public health measures of the twentieth century are linked to our coincident experiences of industrialization, urbanization, and now, the graying of our populations. Each of these developments exposed our fragile bodies to fearsome change, whether professional, geographic, or geriatric. The response in the United States, as in France, has been to seek health security where it makes most sense—from the collective. Early on, workers sought health security in fraternal orders and mutual aid societies. By mid-century, for U.S. workers with steady jobs in certain sectors of the economy, the collective meant private, voluntary employment-based health insurance. Yet now that avenue of socializing the risk of ill health is narrowing by the day.

The relentless rise in medical care costs has led to a dramatic reversal in the spread of employment-based coverage. Rising numbers of uninsured workers are swelling Medicaid roles just as the United States is about to face a tidal wave of retirees who, having completed their professional lives, will lose their employment-based coverage. Not only will they become Medicare beneficiaries; if early indications are correct, many of them will also require Medicaid to finance both their nursing home care and expensive end-of-life medical interventions. The result is a U.S. health care system whose financing will increasingly "go public," in the absence of any policy change, even beyond the massive public subsidies already provided to employer group policies through tax deductions.[1] Hence, the question, properly phrased, is not whether the United States should "go public" or "remain private," it is what role the state should play in directing the mixed public-private system we have been building for nearly a century.

That brings us to a second and related misconception hindering productive debate over the future of U.S. health care: the notion of a "health care market." We saw repeatedly that market forces have had little to do with health care change over the last century. Health care is far too laden with powerful medical professionals, statutory practice barriers, provider networks (which often constitute de facto regional monopolies), oligopolistic pharmaceutical and medical device firms, union power, employer lobbies, and third-party insurance payers. Together, they so warp competitive pressures as to make any sort of market unworkable, at least in the sense that most citizens or their elected officials would recognize. To compare selecting a health care provider to buying a car is to ignore the tremendous concentration of economic power and professional influence on the health care supply side. It also ignores the inherent deleterious effects of serious illness and advanced age, which account for the vast majority of our health care dollars. Such conditions hamper even the most forethoughtful individuals backed by the most supportive families, let alone the vast majority of the population, from exercising anything close to "consumer decision making" for medical care.

The phenomenal rise of HMOs in the 1980s and 1990s can hardly be linked to consumers demanding more group medical practices. On the contrary, the spread of HMOs sparked a consumer rebellion that was embodied in the movement for a "patient's bill of rights," that is, government regulation. The development of managed care was propelled not by health care consumers but by employers who wanted to squelch galloping health care inflation. Moreover, the advent of managed care in the United States has done little to make the price of provider services more transparent to patients, a key indicator of a working market. President Nixon's 1973 HMO Act, which made possible the managed care revolution, undercut one professional monopoly (fee-for-service medicine backed by physicians) in favor of a corporate oligopoly (backed by managed care insurers and employers). Yet now even that new paradigm is unraveling as health care inflation continues apace and more employers reduce or abandon coverage altogether. In the debate over how to fix U.S. health care, the massive imperfections of the "health care market" must be explicitly addressed. Market forces should never be portrayed as some sort of invisible hand that will automatically lead to efficient and just outcomes.[2] Even more important, Americans should ask whether the ideal of price transparency for patients should also be applied to the management of the nation's health care resources. Perhaps insurers, hospitals, and health professionals who had to answer to the people and their representatives would be more efficient with our health care dollars. And where tough decisions of resource allocation must be made, those who make them should be democratically accountable to the citizens whose lives and prosperity are at stake. To take such a stand is surely polemical, but at least it responds to the relevant question: What role should our government play in directing the United States' public-private health care system?

France also suffers from misconceptions regarding the history of its health care system that hinder reasoned consideration of potential solutions. In fact, in the same way that suspiciously un-American qualities are embedded in the popular U.S. conception of "socialized medicine," "managed care" in France is anxiously regarded as an insidious undermining of "la civilisation française" under which patient choice and physicians' clinical freedoms are paramount. Just as many Americans acquired their dark view of national health insurance during the cold war, when AMA propagandists equated it with Communist tyranny, many French now associate managed care with a brutal U.S. social model and the mindless pressures of economic globalization.

It is not that the French fear private insurers or providers. After all, throughout the twentieth century France has enthusiastically embraced a far larger private health care sector than many of its European neighbors and Canada. Indeed, the French experience with mutual aid societies, their patronage of Europe's largest private hospital sector, their overwhelming insistence on private ambulatory care practitioners, as well as their widespread enrollment in private supplemental health coverage all testify to the nation's favorable history with private medical care and health security.

It is that managed care techniques—or any plan for that matter—that would dethrone *Sécurité Sociale* and threaten the realm of private fee-for-service medicine is immediately portrayed as a traitorous abandonment of the French social model. This is not to say that the French public should not maintain a healthy skepticism about adopting managed care approaches from the United States, whose health care system is demonstrably less equitable and far more costly. But to reject managed care techniques out of hand is debilitating. Again, just as in the United States, it is not simply a question of private or public control, but rather of the role the state should play in regulating France's mixed public-private health care system.[3]

One place to seek out whether managed care can work in France is *Sécurité Sociale* itself. Recent reforms have made gatekeeping primary care physicians from whom a patient must obtain a referral before seeing a specialist increasingly widespread and accepted. Confidentiality rules have also been bent with the issuance of new electronically coded *Sécurité Sociale* cards, allowing physicians online access to a patient's medical chart. Other reforms have spread physicians' use of scientifically determined practice regimens known as "best practices."[4] But if these reforms demonstrate the potential of *Sécurité Sociale* to innovate a sort of "state-led managed care" that is more democratic and transparent than its U.S. counterpart, France remains beholden to powerful vested interests and outdated conceptions of health care financing, which threaten the nation's economic stability. In both France and the United States, doctors, employers, workers' unions, and insurers have played historical roles in the development of medical care and health security. Through open debates over health system change, both nations must reexamine the historical preeminence granted to each of these actors.

In their quest to bolster professional sovereignty, U.S. and French doctors so mythologized their role in medical care that it now stands in the way of fruitful reform. At the beginning of the twentieth century, physicians were locked in battle with healers and practitioners of various abilities, all claiming to have various curative powers. Through their successful control and application of scientific advancements, allopathic doctors leapt ahead of their rivals, emerging as one of the world's most prestigious and lucrative professions in a remarkably short time. In their battle for professional sovereignty over the course of the century, doctors repeatedly used their corporate political power for material gain. In so doing, physicians perpetuated a cultural conception of "doctor as priest" and of their profession as somehow above the political battles in which they were, in fact, deeply mired. The AMA's long-standing opposition to public health insurance foreclosed successive opportunities for U.S. workers to achieve widespread health security. This past must be squarely confronted, even though many U.S. doctors now serve another master, namely, the managed care corporations on whose provider networks so many of them depend.

French physicians ultimately proved less disruptive to their fellow citizens' pursuit of health security. They nonetheless occasionally used their status as trusted professionals to block discussions over viable reforms and used a "doctor as seer" rhetoric similar to that of their U.S. counterparts to fallaciously stand above the political fray. As debates over health care reform proceed in both nations, the myth of the all-knowing physician must be set aside. In its place, medical models should be considered that use diverse practitioners, including nurses, primary care and specialist physicians, nurse practitioners, certified nurse-midwives, physical therapists, and mental health professionals, to name just the most obvious—all of whom work collaboratively for the good of the individual patient and community health.[5] Such models would be far more effective at combating the fantasy that medicine can cure everything, which has fueled endless expenditures for cures rather than more productive attention to managing chronic illnesses, taking preventive measures, and promoting public health.[6] Patients' new understanding of their bodies and new insights by health care professionals are a vital antidote to twentieth-century mistakes and an imperative response to the twenty-first-century pursuit of health, which has become akin to the quest for the fountain of youth.

Finally, the single most imperative reform to U.S. and French health care is to sever the obsolete link between employment and health security. Whether it is through specific employers (as in the United States) or through financing (as in France), employment-based health care has long outlived its usefulness and stands in the way of economic prosperity and social justice. Today in the United States, it excludes millions merely because of their position in the labor force, especially in small businesses and the service sector, where group coverage is either not available or is prohibitively expensive as a result of insurers' segmentation of the market based on risk class. After the Second World War, U.S. labor leaders and employers extracted what we can now see were short-term gains from insurers by participating in experience-rated insurance. They effectively erected "silos of solidarity," which inevitably took precedence over broader coalitions that would have favored more universal solutions to health security.[7] Now, as the floodwaters rise around them, the silos will not long offer the security that their occupants were once promised. The workers at General Motors are the most notable victims of the deluge, but others cannot help but follow.[8]

In fact, employment-based health security in the United States was built on the same unsustainable ground as France's nineteenth-century system of mutual aid societies. Exclusion and the segmentation of workers by risk and experience are central to its being. In France, the social and economic upheaval of the First World War reoriented the nation toward compulsory, community-rated insurance for industrial workers. This critical juncture set the country on a path toward a system of inclusive, universal health insurance. Now, in the United States, the decline of the manufacturing sector, spiraling health care inflation, an aging labor force, and global economic pressures are delivering a comparable shock. Only by sharing the risk of ill health more broadly, outlawing the segmentation of insurance markets by risk, can Americans avoid an increasingly social Darwinist society wherein the wealthy and healthy enjoy the lion's share of the most technologically advanced health care system in the world.

Although France moved decidedly away from purely employer-specific health security, which is still common in the United States, French union leaders and employers still exert an influence over *Sécurité Sociale* that is out of all proportion to what should be a democratically accountable institution of universal health coverage. This combination of political power and vested interests has resulted in a *France bloquée* on several occasions in recent years, not just on health care but also on pension and employment reform. Moreover, to the extent that *Sécurité Sociale* benefits have been trimmed for budgetary reasons, it has encouraged the spread of private employment-based supplemental insurance among the better paid, thereby undermining health care equality.

In both nations, today's continued link between the workplace and health security is akin to summertime breaks for schools. In the same way that summer breaks once permitted children to help on the family farm in an agricultural economy, employment-based insurance is a relic of a once-dominant industrial economy. In the United States, as the price of health care has climbed, small businesses, the self-employed, and service sectors with less commitment to providing health security have been unable (or unwilling) to adhere to a model developed in the industrial world of the early twentieth century. Based on similar precedents, France's *Sécurité Sociale* has preserved a financial link (through wage levies) to health security because of the once-important might of industrial unions and the role played by occupationally organized mutual aid societies. We can now see that the financing and administration of *Sécurité Sociale* is an artifact of a mid-twentieth-century compromise that effectively healed a nation sharply divided by class and the German occupation. Yet it is now failing to respond to twenty-first century problems.

Today, leaders of virtually every political stripe in both nations advocate more flexible and highly trained workforces to run entrepreneurial firms that can compete in a fast-moving, information-based global economy. This is hardly the world in which employment-based health security was created. To cling to it now is to be enslaved to a past that has clearly outlived its usefulness, and such inflexibility will almost certainly lead to needless suffering and financial hardships for individuals and the gutting of public budgets.

Only if the link between health care financing and security from the calculations of workers and employers is severed will health care cease to hinder employment and economic growth. France's health-related *Sécurité Sociale* wage levies and the United States' even heavier payroll-financed health insurance premiums should be replaced by progressive income taxes. This approach would unleash the skills and productivity of labor forces in both nations by removing barriers to labor mobility and stimulating higher employment rates. U.S. workers would be freed from "job lock," a growing malignancy in the U.S. labor market that forces workers not to seek the best match between their skills and jobs but instead to remain in (or take) jobs that provide health security for them or their family members. In France, the reliance on wage levies to pay for climbing health care costs puts a heavy drag on economic growth, public budgets, and employment, because high compulsory nonwage labor costs dissuade the hiring of new workers.

Moreover, the replacement of payroll levies with a progressive income tax would result in greater equity in the financing of health care. The break-throughs in medical science and related technologies during the twentieth century have led to fantastic gains in quality of life and life expectancy in both nations. Yet these gains, which no one wants to see reversed, are exceedingly expensive. By maintaining health care's financial dependence on wages, the United States and France are in essence carrying forward a nineteenth-century practice. At that time, some workers were able to give up a modicum of their cash wages to protect themselves from the risk of illness or accident, using various types of private mutual aid societies, benefit associations, or fraternal orders. Let us also recall, however, that in the nineteenth century, even in the event of serious illness or accident, medical expenses were typically dwarfed by the value of lost wages. Now the reverse is true. Yet we continue to rely on employers and workers to foot much of the bill for a marvelous but extremely expensive health care infrastructure and its accompanying medical personnel. Thus, even if na-tional prosperity were not at stake, social justice demands a more equitable cost sharing of twenty-first-century health care through a progressive tax that affects not only wages but other sorts of income, profits, and rents.

Obviously, the recommendations outlined above would require signifi-cant reforms to U.S. and French health care. They would change how each nation pays for and administers health insurance, even reformulating the very nature of insurers and their relationship to government. For private-practice medicine, however, an ideal long shared by the Americans and the French, the effect of such major reforms would be salutary. If nothing else, the history of French health care (and Medicare) demonstrates that a larger role for public insurers need not diminish the clinical freedoms of practi-tioners or patients' freedom of choice among them. In fact, the statutory protections enjoyed by French physicians repeatedly protected their diag-nostic and therapeutic freedoms, while U.S. doctors, for all their political might, lost much of their sovereignty over medical decision making, even as their patients were confined to provider networks.

Even if the major reforms that our reckoning with the past seems to advise prove impossible to realize, smaller changes in health care could also be consequential. Certainly, few of the proponents of France's 1930 compulsory health insurance law for industrial workers dreamed that it would one day serve as a starting point for the universal coverage achieved in 2000. Historians made that connection with their narratives. Between them lay myriad tweaks and changes, some that strengthened and expanded health coverage, others that weakened it, and still others that wrought great progress, such as the founding of *Sécurité Sociale* in 1945. But even in that turbulent year of reform, when it seemed that all was possible, France preserved the link between wage levies and health insurance, and reaffirmed its protections of private-practice fee-for-service medicine.

The history of U.S. health care has followed a similar pattern. Occasional major reforms punctuate longer periods during which underlying causes such as tax laws, medical science, and other seemingly small adjustments have together led to substantial developments. To make this observation is not to advocate indifference. Far from it. Rather, it is to say that health care reformers must live in their own eras, that incremental reforms can add up to very big change, as long as they are well informed by historical experience and based on a broad consideration of all possibilities. What is most important is not the breadth of reform: that will be determined by the larger historical context of the moment. It is whom the reform is designed to help—historically entrenched interests or growing portions of the nation's citizenry who suffer from health insecurity.

My family and I often vacation in the Pacific Northwest where we have a cabin on Mount Hood, just 45 minutes from Portland. Sitting in my favorite diner on the mountain, reading the local newspaper, I came across the following letter to the editor: "I am your mail carrier, Dana Vedder. My son Dakota needs three surgeries, but we do not have health insurance. If anybody would like to make a donation for his medical treatment, they can go to the Clackamas County Bank and make a deposit to the account for Dana Vedder. Thank you!" An editor's note followed, explaining that five-year-old Dakota, "a cute little kid," suffers from a severe hearing impairment. Despite the Vedder family's forty-six years of delivering the mail on Mount Hood, as private contractors they enjoy no health coverage from the U.S. Postal Service.[9] Needless to say, Dakota's condition is uninsurable through an individual policy. I had alighted from a plane not ten hours before, en route from a comparably rural region in southern France where the Vedders' plight could not have been imagined. Yet here the tragedy seemed accepted as if little could be done about it, except the Vedders' appeal for charity, a courageous step that many similarly afflicted families might refuse to take. Why is it, I wondered, that U.S. political leaders—who must know that such problems were long ago solved in so many other countries—care so little about Dakota Vedder and the countless others like him?

A political cartoon during the Clinton health care reform debate of 1994 rightly mocked the U.S. political class and the media when it observed that politicians and news commentators repeatedly dismissed reform options based solely on whether they were "politically viable." Never mind that the public never heard the logic behind, or the evidence for or against, the option in question so that the political class could test its viability. Political leaders were so determined "to do nothing that wasn't just and right," as John Maynard Keynes once observed of Woodrow Wilson, that nothing was done at all.[10] That is another way of saying that inaction in the face of today's health care crises is an irresponsibly radical position.

NOTES

1 Common Ideals, Divergent Nations

1. Marc Bloch, "Pour une histoire comparée des sociétés européennes," *Revue de Synthèse Historique* 46 (1928): 15–50.

2. For more on Enlightenment ideals in the United States and France, see Mark Hulliung, *Citizens and Citoyens: Republicans and Liberals in America and France* (Cambridge, MA: Harvard University Press, 2002); Patrice Higonnet, *Sister Republics: The Origins of French and American Republicanism* (Cambridge, MA: Harvard University Press, 1988); Joseph Klaits and Michael H. Haltzel, eds., *Liberty/Liberté: The American and French Experiences* (Washington, DC: Woodrow Wilson Center Press, 1991).

3. Kaiser Family Foundation, "Distribution of Out-of-Pocket Expenditures on Health Care Services," Health Care Snapshot (Kaiser Family Foundation, 2003); Robert P. Hartwig, "What's Behind the Rising Cost of Auto and Homeowner's Insurance," (Insurance Information Institute, 2003), www.iii.org/media/hottopics/hot/20022003outlook/; Béatrice Majnoni d'Intignano and Philippe Ulman, *Economie de la santé* (Paris: Presses Universitaires de France, 2001), 299; Paul V. Dutton and Bruno Valat, "La réforme de l'assurance maladie aux Etats-Unis et en France, 1993–2004," *Histoire et Sociétés: Revue Européenne d'Histoire Sociale* 11 (July 2004): 49–63.

4. Jean de Kervasdoué and Victor Rodwin, "La politique de santé et le rôle de l'Etat, 1945–1980," in *La santé rationnée?* ed. Jean de Kervasdoué, John Kimberly, and Victor Rodwin (Paris: Economica, 1981), 23.

5. "The President's Page," *Journal of the American Medical Association* (hereafter *JAMA*), 24 February 1951, 567.

6. *OECD Health Data 2006* (Paris: Organization for Economic Cooperation and Development, 2006), www.ecosante.org/oecd.htm; Stephen Heffler et al., "US Health Spending Projections for 2004–2014," *Health Affairs*, Web exclusive, 23 February 2005, www.healthaffairs.org/WebExclusives.php.

7. U.S. Census Bureau press release, 29 August 2006, www.census.gov/Press-Release/www/releases/archives/income_wealth/007419.html; World Health Organization, *World Health Report 2000*, 21 June 2001, statistical annex, 152–55; Ichiro Kawachi, "Why the United States Is Not Number One in Health," in *Healthy, Wealthy, and Fair: Health Care and the Good Society*, ed. James A. Morone and Lawrence Jacobs (New York: Oxford University Press, 2005), 19–36; Jean de Kervasdoué, ed., *Le carnet de santé de la France en 2000* (Paris: Fédération Nationale de la Mutualité Française, 2000), 76.

8. "In the 5 Largest European Countries, French Health Care System Most Popular at Home and Most Admired Abroad," *Health Care News*, 29 July 2004, 1–3; "Public's Assessment

of the State of the U.S. Health Care System," *Kaiser Health Poll Report* (January–February 2004).

9. Victor G. Rodwin, "The Rise of Managed Care in the United States: Lessons for French Health Policy," in *Health Policy Reform, National Schemes and Globalization,* ed. C. Altenstetter and J. Björkman (New York: St. Martins, 1997), 55–58.

10. De Kervasdoué, ed., *Le carnet de santé de la France* 62, 76; Blue Cross Blue Shield, *Medical Cost Reference Guide* (2004), 8; Alain Bourrez, "Le contrôle interne de la dépense dans la branche maladie," in *La maîtrise des dépenses de santé en Europe et en Amérique du Nord,* ed. Etienne Douat (Rennes: Université de Rennes, 1996), 331–34.

11. Yves Poirmeur, "L'affichage de la politique de maîtrise des dépenses de santé dans les programmes de J. Chirac, E. Balladur et L. Jospin pour la campagne pour l'élection présidentielle de 1995," in Douat, ed., *La maîtrise des dépenses de santé,* 71–89.

12. Jerome P. Kassirer, *On the Take: How Medicine's Complicity with Big Business Can Endanger Your Health* (New York: Oxford University Press, 2005), 131–44; David Dranove, *The Economic Evolution of American Health Care: From Marcus Welby to Managed Care* (Princeton, NJ: Princeton University Press, 2000), 86–90, 136–58.

13. Ruth Berins Collier and David Collier, *Shaping the Political Arena: Critical Junctures, the Labor Movement, and Regime Dynamics in Latin America* (Princeton, NJ: Princeton University Press, 1991).

14. Margaret Levi, "A Model, a Method, and a Map: Rational Choice in Comparative Historical Analysis," in *Comparative Politics: Rationality, Culture, and Structure,* ed. Mark I. Lichbach and Alan S. Zuckerman (Cambridge, U.K.: Cambridge University Press, 1997), as cited by Paul Pierson, "Increasing Returns, Path Dependence and the Study of Politics," *American Political Science Review* 94, 2 (June 2000): 252. See also Paul Pierson, *Politics in Time: History, Institutions, and Social Analysis* (Princeton, NJ: Princeton University Press, 2004).

15. Rosemary Stevens, *American Medicine and the Public Interest* (Berkeley: University of California Press, 1998), 528–29.

16. Alexis de Tocqueville, *Journey to America,* ed. J. P. Mayer, trans. George Lawrence (New York: Anchor, 1971), 149 (notation of 1 October 1831).

17. Willard Sterne Randall, *Thomas Jefferson: A Life* (New York: Harper, 1993), 213, 300–303; Fergus M. Bordewich, *Bound for Canaan: The Underground Railroad and the War for the Soul of America* (New York: Harper Collins, 2005), 194.

18. Jean-Jacques Rousseau, *The Social Contract,* trans. Maurice Cranston (New York: Penguin, 1981), 69–78.

19. Michael K. Brown, *Race, Money and the American Welfare State* (Ithaca, NY: Cornell University Press, 1999), 17. See also Robert C. Lieberman, *Shifting the Color Line: Race and the American Welfare State* (Cambridge, MA: Harvard University Press, 1998).

20. Paul V. Dutton, *Origins of the French Welfare State: The Struggle for Social Reform in France, 1914–1947* (New York: Cambridge University Press, 2002), 5, 39, 220–21; Colin Gordon, *Dead on Arrival: The Politics of Health Care in Twentieth-Century America* (Princeton, NJ: Princeton University Press, 2003), 7; Alan Derickson, *Health Security for All: Dreams of Universal Health Care in America* (Baltimore: Johns Hopkins University Press, 2005), chap. 5. See also Elinor Accampo, Rachel G. Fuchs, and Mary Lynn Stewart, *Gender and the Politics of Social Reform* (Baltimore: Johns Hopkins University Press, 1995); Gwendolyn Mink, "The Lady and the Tramp: Gender, Race, and the Origins of the American Welfare State," in *Women, the State, and Welfare,* ed. Linda Gordon (Madison: University of Wisconsin Press, 1990).

21. Timothy Smith, *France in Crisis: Welfare, Inequality and Globalization since 1980* (Cambridge, U.K.: Cambridge University Press, 2004), 143–44.

22. Thomas C. Buchmueller and Agnes Couffinhal, "Private Health Insurance in France," *OECD Working Papers 12* 3 (March 2004): 13–15; A. Bocognano et al., "La complémentaire maladie en France: Qui bénéficie de quels remboursements? Résultats de l'enquête Santé Protection Sociale 1998," *Questions d'économie de la santé,* (CREDES, 2000) 32:1–4.

23. U.S. Health and Human Services, Agency for Health Care Research and Quality, *2005 National Health Care Disparities Report,* AHRQ Publication 06-0017, December 2005, 3–4.

24. Consolidated Omnibus Budget Reconciliation Act (COBRA) of 1986; Bureau of Labor Statistics, "Quarterly Data on Business Dynamics by Size of Firm," December 2005, http://www.bls.gov/bdm/.

25. Author's interview with Amy D., 23 May 2006.

26. D. Green et al., *Health Care in France* (London: Civitas, 2005), 1.

27. "La contribution sociale généralisée: Quatorzième rapport au Président de la République (analyse)," 14 June 2005.

28. "France Announces Major Reform Project, Including Overhaul of Income Tax System," *BNA Daily Tax Report,* 2 September 2005.

29. "Small Firms Forge Plans for '06 Health-Care Costs," *Atlanta Business Chronicle,* 25 November 2005; James C. Robinson, "Renewed Emphasis on Consumer Cost Sharing in Health Insurance Benefit Design," *Health Affairs,* 20 March 2002; Gary Claxton et al., "Health Benefits in 2006: Premium Increases Moderate, Enrollment in Consumer-Directed Health Plans Remains Modest," *Health Affairs,* 26 September 2006, doi: 10.1377/hlthaff.25.w476.

30. Zeynep Or, "Improving the Performance of Health Care Systems: From Measures to Action (A Review of Experiences in Four OECD Countries)," OECD, Labour Market and Social Policy Occasional Paper no. 57, 25 January 2002, 31.

31. Assar Lindbeck and Dennis Snower, "The Insider-Outsider Theory: A Survey," Discussion Paper Series no. 534, Forschungsinstitut zur Zukunft der Arbeit, July 2002.

32. Interview with Jean-Philippe Cotis, Chief Economist, Organization for Economic Co-operation and Development (OECD), *Le monde,* 30 March 2006.

33. Jonathan Gruber and Brigitte C. Madrian, "Health Insurance, Labor Supply, and Job Mobility: A Critical Review of the Literature," Working Paper 8817, National Bureau of Economic Research, March 2002.

34. Ibid., 28–29.

35. "Rising Cost of Health Benefits Cited as Factor in Slump of Jobs," *New York Times,* 19 August 2004.

36. Wal-Mart Stores Inc., "Supplemental Benefits Documentation," Benefits Strategy, Board of Directors Retreat FYO6, 14.

37. Kaiser Family Foundation, *Employer Health Benefits,* 2005 Summary of Findings; Paul Krugman and Robin Wells, "The Health Care Crisis and What to Do About It," *New York Review of Books,* 23 March 2006.

38. Todd Gilmer and Richard Kronick, "It's the Premiums, Stupid: Projections of the Uninsured through 2013," *Health Affairs,* 5 April 2005, Web exclusive, doi 10.1377hlthaff.W5.143.

39. Letter from Douglas Holtz-Eakin, Director of the Congressional Budget Office, to Joe Barton, Chair of the House Committee on Energy and Commerce, 4 March 2005.

40. John Sheils and Randall Haught, "The Cost of Tax-Exempt Health Benefits in 2004," *Health Affairs*, 25 February 2004, doi: 10.1377/hlthaff.W4.106.

41. Capitation is a form of compensation whereby doctors are prepaid on a per capita basis to provide a specified package of services to a defined group of patients. It is commonly used by managed care organizations to create a financial incentive for physicians to deliver cost-efficient services.

42. Victor G. Rodwin, "Health Care Reform in France—The Birth of State-Led Managed Care," *New England Journal of Medicine,* 25 November 2004, 2259–62.

43. Claude Le Pen, "Vers une culture de l'évaluation économique des produits de santé?" *Réalités industrielles—Annales des Mines,* 22 June 2005, 36–39.

44. George Rosen, *The Structure of American Medical Practice, 1875–1941* (Philadelphia: University of Pennsylvania Press, 1983); Pierre Guillaume, *Le rôle social du médecin depuis deux siècles, 1800–1945* (Paris: Association pour l'Etude de l'histoire de la Sécurité Sociale, 1996).

45. Jonathan E. Fielding and Pierre-Jean Lancry, "Lessons from France—'Vive la Différence,'" *JAMA,* 11 August 1993, 749.

46. Rosemary Stevens, *In Sickness and in Wealth: American Hospitals in the Twentieth Century* (Baltimore: Johns Hopkins University Press, 1999).

47. Victor G. Rodwin, "The Health Care System under French National Health Insurance: Lessons for Health Reform in the United States," *American Journal of Public Health* 93, 1 (January 2003): 31–37.

48. "Summary of Findings: Privatization of Public Hospitals," prepared for the Henry J. Kaiser Family Foundation by the Economic and Social Research Institute, January 1999, 5.

49. Bloch, "Pour une histoire comparée des sociétés européennes," 20–28.

50. Bruno Valat, *Histoire de la Sécurité Sociale, 1945–1967: L'Etat, l'institution et la santé* (Paris: Economica, 2001), 171–77.

51. Daniel M. Fox, *Power and Illness: The Failure and Future of American Health Policy* (Berkeley: University of California Press, 1993), 6.

52. David U. Himmelstein et al., "Illness and Injury as Contributors to Bankruptcy," *Health Affairs*, 2 February 2005, 63–67, doi: 10.1377/hlthaff.w5.63.

2 Health Insurance and the Rise of Private-Practice Medicine, 1915–1930

1. For more on the physicians' clinical gaze, see Michel Foucault, *Naissance de la clinique* (Paris: Presses Universitaires de France, 1963).

2. Alonzo L. Hamby, "Progressivism: A Century of Change and Rebirth," in *Progressivism and the New Democracy*, ed. Sidney M. Milkis and Jerome M. Mileur (Amherst: University of Massachusetts Press, 1999), 41–80; Gary Gerstle, "The Protean Character of American Liberalism," *American Historical Review* 99, 4 (October 1994): 1043–73; Richard L. McCormick, "The Discovery That Business Corrupts Politics: A Reappraisal of the Origins of Progressivism," *American Historical Review* 86, 2 (April 1981): 247–74.

3. Daniel T. Rodgers, *Atlantic Crossings: Social Politics in a Progressive Age* (Cambridge, MA: Harvard University Press, 1998), 52–59.

4. Hamby, "Progressivism," 47–48.

5. Beatrix Hoffman, *The Wages of Sickness: The Politics of Health Insurance in Progressive America* (Chapel Hill: University of North Carolina Press, 2001), 25.

6. Bentley B. Gilbert, *The Evolution of National Insurance in Britain: The Origins of the Welfare State* (London: Joseph, 1966); testimony before the Ohio Health and Old Age Insurance Commission, "Health, Health Insurance, Old Age Pensions: Report, Recommendations, Dissenting Opinions" (Columbus, OH: F. J. Heer, 1919), 180–81.

7. Alfred Cox, "Seven Years of National Health Insurance in England: A Retrospect," *Journal of the American Medical Association* 76 (1921): 1313–14.

8. Committee on Social Insurance, American Association for Labor Legislation, "Health Insurance: Tentative Draft of an Act," *American Labor Legislation Review* (June 1916): 241–42.

9. Ibid., 255–56.

10. Ibid., 248.

11. Ibid., 255–56.

12. B. S. Warren and Edgar Sydenstriker, "Health Insurance, Its Relation to Public Health," *United States Public Health Service Bulletin*, no. 76 (March 1916): 49–50.

13. *American Labor Legislation Review* 7, 1 (1917): 207.

14. Ibid., 211.

15. Chantal Metzger, "Relations entre autonomistes lorrains et alsaciens de 1919 à 1932," 103e Congrès national des sociétés savantes, Nancy-Metz 1978, *Histoire-moderne* 2: 155–70.

16. Alexandre Millerand, *Le retour de l'Alsace-Lorraine à la France* (Paris: Charpentier, 1923), 70–72.

17. "Assurance Maladie en Alsace," *Le Médecin Syndicaliste*, September 1921, 517; Auguste Herrmann, "L'organisation et le mécanisme des assurances sociales d'Alsace-Lorraine," *Le Médecin de l'Alsace et de Lorraine*, 22 October 1922, 231–32; Office Général des Assurances Sociales d'Alsace et de Lorraine, *Les assurances sociales en Alsace et Lorraine*, 2nd edition (Strasbourg, 1922), statistical tables; *L'assurance maladie et les oeuvres sociales dans les industries d'Alsace et de Lorraine* (Metz: Paul Even, 1922), 5–7; transcript of paper delivered by Paul Schlumberger, vice president of the Société Industrielle de Mulhouse, Comité National d'Etudes Sociales et Politiques, 13 January 1930, 15–18.

18. E. Schmidt, annual report of the Secrétariat de la Fédération des Syndicats Médicaux d'Alsace, *Le Médecin de l'Alsace et de Lorraine*, 16 March 1922, 14.

19. Ibid., 142–43.

20. "L'assurance-maladie et les médecins en Alsace," *Le Médecin Syndicaliste* no. 5 (May 1920): 139; "Le contrat collectif: La loi sur l'assurance contre la maladie et les Syndicats des Médecins d'Alsace," *Le Médecin Syndicaliste* no. 6 (June 1920): 173.

21. M. Degas, *Les assurances sociales* (Paris: Dunod, 1924), xv–xvi.

22. Edouard Grinda, *Rapport fait au nom de la Commission d'Assurance et de Prévoyance Sociales chargée d'examiner le projet de loi sur les assurances sociales*, appendix to the minutes of the session of 31 January, no. 5505 (Paris: Imprimerie de la Chambre, 1923), 39.

23. *Revue Politique et Parlementaire,* 10 February and 10 April 1923, cited by A. Rey, *La question des assurances sociales* (Paris: Félix Alcan, 1925), 215.

24. "La loi folle: De nouvelles protestations contre les assurances sociales," *La France Active* 102 (July–August 1929): 49–56.

25. *The Monitor* 3 (March 1917): 18, as quoted by Hoffman, *Wages of Sickness*, 96.

26. Testimony before the Ohio Health and Old Age Insurance Commission, "Health, Health Insurance, Old Age Pensions: Report, Recommendations, Dissenting Opinions" (Columbus, OH: F. J. Heer, 1919), 427.

27. R.-P. Duchemin, letter addressed to the Conseil d'Etat, "La Confédération Générale de la production Française et les Assurances Sociales," reprinted in *Les assurances Sociales* 4 (April 1930): 25–28.

28. Jean-Claude Devinck, "La création de la médecine du travail en France, 1914–1946," Ph.D. diss., Ecole des Hautes Etudes en Sciences Sociales, 2001, 30–44.

29. James H. S. Bossard, "A Sociologist Looks at the Doctors," in *The Medical Profession and the Public: Currents and Counter-Currents* (Philadelphia: American Academy of Political and Social Science, 1934), 1–10, esp. 5; Sanford Jacoby, *Modern Manors: Welfare Capitalism since the New Deal* (Princeton, NJ: Princeton University Press, 1997), 69, 78.

30. Minutes of the Comité National d'Etudes Sociales et Politiques, 13 January 1930, 22.

31. Colin Gordon, *Dead on Arrival: The Politics of Health Care in Twentieth-Century America* (Princeton, NJ: Princeton University Press, 2003), 50–51.

32. Desiré Ley, "Les allocations maladie du Consortium textile de Roubaix-Tourcoing," *Bulletin de la Fédération Nationale des Syndicats Médicaux de France* no. 6 (June 1927): 127–28.

33. Paul Guérin, *L'Etat contre le médecin: Vers une renaissance corporative*, preface by Paul Bourget (Paris: Editions Médicales Norbert Maloine, 1929), 238–39.

34. P. Desrousseaux, "Les assurances sociales: Etat actuel de la question," *Bulletin de la Fédération Nationale des Syndicats Médicaux de France* no. 7 (November 1926): 173.

35. Secretary general's report, *Bulletin de la Fédération Nationale des Syndicats Médicaux de France* no. 6 (October 1926): 149.

36. Indeed, after tortuous negotiations with the Paris doctors' association to provide medical benefits to their workers, industrialists promptly cancelled the contract once it became apparent that compulsory insurance would become law. See "Contrat avec la Caisse de Compensation de la Région Parisienne," *Bulletin Officiel des Médecins de la Seine* no. 6 (June 1927).

37. René Lafontaine, "Etude resumée du contrat de Roubaix-Tourcoing, *Le Médecin Syndicaliste* no. 2 (January 1926): 34.

38. Report of the Assemblée Générale de l'Union des Syndicats Médicaux de France, 4–5 December 1925, *Le Médecin Syndicaliste* no. 7, 1 April 1926.

39. René Lafontaine, "Etude resumée du contrat de Roubaix-Tourcoing, *Le Médecin Syndicaliste* no. 2 (January 1926): 36.

40. Testimony before the Ohio Health and Old Age Insurance Commission, "Health, Health Insurance, Old Age Pensions: Report, Recommendations, Dissenting Opinions" (Columbus, OH: F. J. Heer, 1919), 304.

41. *American Federationist* 23, 11 (November 1916): 1072–74.

42. Testimony before the Ohio Health and Old Age Insurance Commission, "Health, Health Insurance, Old Age Pensions: Report, Recommendations, Dissenting Opinions" (Columbus, OH: F. J. Heer, 1919), 304.

43. New York Senate Judiciary hearing, 7 March 1917, American Association of Labor Legislation Papers, microfilm edition (Glen Rock, NJ, 1974), reel 62, as quoted by Hoffman, *Wages of Sickness*, 123.

44. *American Labor Legislation Review* 9, 1 (1919): 162.

45. *L'Humanité*, 11 June 1923.

46. Perrot, rapporteur, CGT general assembly, cited by A. Rey, *La question des assurances sociales*, 384–85.

47. "Topics of the Month," *Fraternal Monitor,* 1 December 1907, 13, as quoted by David T. Beito, *From Mutual Aid to the Welfare State: Fraternal Societies and Social Services, 1890–1967* (Chapel Hill: University of North Carolina Press, 2000), 144.

48. "Menace of Social Insurance," *Fraternal Monitor,* 1 November 1919, 8, as quoted by Beito, *From Mutual Aid to the Welfare State*, 152.

49. Henry Rosenfeld, "Life Insurance as a Factor in the Solution of Sociological Problems," Rosenfeld papers, file 9, box 58A (1912), as quoted by Jennifer Klein, *For All These*

Rights: Business, Labor, and the Shaping of America's Public-Private Welfare State (Princeton, NJ: Princeton University Press, 2003), 21.

50. Klein, *For All These Rights,* 33.

51. Report of the Committee on Social Insurance, presented to the National Fraternal Congress of America, Chicago, 31 August 1921, National Civic Federation Papers, box 69, as quoted by Hoffman, *Wages of Sickness,* 106.

52. Hoffman, *Wages of Sickness,* 36, 108.

53. Frederick L. Hoffman, "Some Fallacies of Compulsory Health Insurance," *Scientific Monthly* 4, 4 (April 1917): 306–16, esp. 306–7, 309.

54. Ibid., 307.

55. Letter from Henri Vermont to the Conseil Supérieur des Sociétés de Secours Mutuels, *Bulletin des Sociétés des Secours Mutuels* (September 1921): 133–36; Henri Vermont, "La loi des assurances sociales," *La Réforme Sociale* (January 1922): 10–34, esp. 29. Also see Yannick Marec, "L'apôtre de la mutualité: Henri Vermont, 1836–1928," *L'Economie Sociale* (January 1987): 3–39.

56. These included Senator Paul Strauss and Deputy Gaston Roussel. See Jean Bennet, *Biographes de personalités mutualistes, XIXe et XXe siècles* (Paris: Mutualité Française, 1987), 341, 401–4, 444.

57. *Bulletin Officiel de la Fédération Nationale de la Mutualité Française* (hereafter FNMF) 32 (September–December 1926): 44.

58. For examples, see "Une grande conférence de M. Georges Petit sur les assurances sociales" and "Lettre de M. Georges Petit à M. le Sénateur Chauveau," *FNMF* 31 (May–August 1926): 2–5.

59. Report on the Assemblée Générale of the Syndicat des Médecins de la Seine, 21 June 1925, *Bulletin du Syndicat des Médecins de la Seine* no. 9 (September 1925): 231.

60. For an excellent account of the French medical profession in the nineteenth century, see Alexander F. Dracobly, "Disciplining the Doctor: Medical Morality and Professionalism in Nineteenth-Century France," Ph.D. diss., University of Chicago, 1997. Also see Jacques Léonard, *La médecine entre les savoirs et les pouvoirs: Histoire intellectuelle et politique de la médecine française au XIXe siècle* (Paris: Aubier-Montaigne, 1981); Jack D. Ellis, *The Physician-Legislators of France: Medicine and Politics in the Early Third Republic, 1870–1914* (Cambridge, U.K.: Cambridge University Press, 1990).

61. Ronald Numbers, *Almost Persuaded* (Baltimore: Johns Hopkins University Press, 1978), 26–29.

62. *Journal of the American Medical Association* (hereafter *JAMA*) 54 (1910): 225–26, as quoted by Numbers, *Almost Persuaded,* 33, 37.

63. René Lafontaine, "Comment se présente pour les médecins le problème de l'Assurance maladie," *Le Médecin Syndicaliste* no. 9 (September 1920): 238–40, italics in the original.

64. As quoted by Numbers, *Almost Persuaded,* 75.

65. William P. Cunningham, "A Bolshevik Bolus," *New York Medical Journal* 108 (1918): 1061–65, as quoted by Numbers, *Almost Persuaded,* 88.

66. *Pennsylvania Medical Journal* 22 (1918): 62; Numbers, *Almost Persuaded,* 77.

67. Testimony before the Ohio Health and Old Age Insurance Commission, "Health, Health Insurance, Old Age Pensions: Report, Recommendations, Dissenting Opinions" (Columbus, OH: F. J. Heer, 1919), 195.

68. For more on the German influence on France's debate concerning social reform, see Allan Mitchell, *The Divided Path: The German Influence on Social Reform in France after 1870* (Chapel Hill: University of North Carolina Press, 1991), chaps. 6 and 11.

69. Report on the Assemblée Générale of the Syndicat des Médecins de la Seine, 4 December 1921, *Bulletin Officiel du Syndicat des Médecins de la Seine*, nos. 1–2 (January–February 1922): 21. Jayle's argument against health insurance resembles that of the American Medical Association. See "The 'Health Rate' of a Nation," *JAMA*, 1 February 1919, 346–47.

70. Report on the Assemblée Générale of the Union des Syndicats Médicaux de France, 9–11 December 1921, *Le Médecin Syndicaliste*, no. 1 (January 1922): 52.

71. See Mitchell, *The Divided Path*, 130–32, 261–75.

72. See, for example, E. Wennagel, "Impressions de l'Assemblée générale de l'USMF," *Le Médecin d'Alsace et de Lorraine*, 1 February 1924, 65–69.

73. Agenda of the Assemblée Générale, 8 May 1927, *Bulletin Officiel du Syndicat des Médecins de la Seine* no. 5 (May 1927): 123.

74. Numbers, *Almost Persuaded*, 38.

75. Bureau of Labor Statistics, *Proceedings of the Conference on Social Insurance*, 5–9 December 1916, Bulletin no. 212, (Washington: Government Printing Office, 1917), 717–19; *New York State Medical Journal* 16 (1916): 202, as quoted in Numbers, *Almost Persuaded*, 38, 50–51.

76. This dynamic had already exhibited itself in the late nineteenth century. See Martha L. Hildreth, "Medical Rivalries and Medical Politics: The French Physicians' Union Movement and the Medical Assistance Law of 1893," *Journal of the History of Medicine and Allied Sciences* 42 (1987): 5–29.

77. Paul Starr, *The Social Transformation of American Medicine* (New York: Basic Books, 1982), 253.

78. Report of Work, AALL, 1921, reel 61, as quoted by Hoffman, *Wages of Sickness*, 178.

79. *Bulletin Officiel du Syndicat des Médecins de la Seine*, no. 1 (January 1928): 26–27.

80. Paul Cibrie, *Syndicalisme médical* (Paris: Confédération des Syndicats Médicaux Français, 1954), 70.

81. Ibid., 83.

82. Report on the XVe Congrès National de la Mutualité Française, *FNMF* 43 (May–June 1930): 4–7.

83. *Le Matin*, 26 April 1930; *Les Assurances Sociales* (July 1930): 28. See also *FNMF* 43 (May–June 1930): 23.

84. Minutes of the House of Delegates, *JAMA* 74 (1920): 1319.

3 Health Security, the State, and Civil Society, 1930–1940

1. On interwar social welfare, see Paul V. Dutton, *Origins of the French Welfare State: The Struggle for Social Reform in France, 1914–1947* (New York: Cambridge University Press, 2002).

2. Daniel T. Rodgers, *Atlantic Crossings: Social Politics in a Progressive Age* (Cambridge, MA: Harvard University Press, 1998), 437–42.

3. Georges Duhamel, "Les excès de l'Etatisme et les responsabilités de la médecine," *Revue des Deux Mondes*, 15 May 1934, 278–84.

4. Jennifer Klein, *For All These Rights, Business, Labor, and the Shaping of America's Public-Private Welfare State* (Princeton, NJ: Princeton University Press, 2003), 119; Christian Maillard, *Histoire de l'hôpital de 1940 à nos jours* (Paris: Bordas, 1988), 7.

5. The six foundations were the Carnegie Foundation, the Josiah Macy, Jr. Foundation, the Milbank Memorial Fund, the Russell Sage Foundation, the Twentieth Century Fund, and

the Julius Rosenwald Fund. See Odin Anderson, *Health Services as a Growth Enterprise in the United States Since 1875*, 2nd ed. (Ann Arbor, MI: Health Administration Press, 1990), 97.

6. *Medical Care for the American People: The Final Report of the Committee on the Costs of Medical Care*, as adopted 31 October 1932 (Chicago: University of Chicago Press, 1938; repr. Arno Press, 1972), 81.

7. Klein, *For All These Rights*, 124; Susan Smith, *Sick and Tired of Being Sick and Tired: Black Women's Health Activism in America, 1890–1950* (Philadelphia: University of Pennsylvania Press, 1995).

8. Klein, *For All These Rights*, 122–25.

9. *Medical Care for the American People*, 109.

10. Ibid., 131.

11. Ibid., 169.

12. Ibid., 160.

13. Ibid., 179.

14. Health insurance funds commonly entered into contracts with a variety of *syndicats médicaux*, including those of surgeons, dentists, midwives, and pharmacists.

15. Minutes of the Assemblée Générale de la Confédération des Syndicats Médicaux Français, 19 December 1937, reported in *Le Médecin de France*, 1 March 1938, 220. See also see *Le Médecin de France* (March–April 1946): 267–69.

16. Romain Laveille, *Histoire de la mutualité* (Paris: Hachette, 1964), 117.

17. *Journal Officiel de la République Française*, laws and decrees, 1 May 1930, 4821.

18. Pierre Guillaume, *Mutualistes et médecins: Conflits et convergences XIXe–XXe siècles* (Paris: La Mutualité Française, 2000), 137.

19. Commentary by Léon Heller, president of the Fédération Nationale de la Mutualité Française, *Le Matin*, 14 April 1932.

20. *Le Médecin de France*, 26 January, 100.

21. "Note sur les oeuvres sociales mutualistes diverses," Centres des Archives Contemporaines (hereafter CAC), dossier 1990 0604/7.

22. "Médecine générale, rapport par Jean Basset," report to the Sixteenth National Congress of the Mutualité Française, 1933, 33.

23. Leaders of the Confédération des Syndicats Médicaux Français reported the most egregious violations of the medical charter by mutual society social insurance funds in *Le Médecin de France*, 1 January 1932, 25; 26 January 1932, 97–105; 12 February 1932, 133–43; letter from Léon Heller, president of the Fédération Nationale de la Mutualité Française, to Camille Chautemps, prime minister, 16 July 1937, Archives Nationales de France (hereafter AN), box F60 651. See also Paul Marcadé, *Le médecin français et la loi sur les assurances sociales* (Bordeaux: Imprimerie-Librarie de l'Université, 1933), 66–72.

24. *Le Médecin de France*, November 1931, as quoted by Guillaume, *Mutualistes et médecins*, 149.

25. *Le Médecin de France*, 18 April 1932, 365–67.

26. Ibid., 2 May 1932, 403.

27. Ibid., 10 May 1932, 457.

28. Pierre Guillaume, *Le rôle du médecin depuis deux siècles, 1800–1945* (Paris: Association pour l'Etude de l'histoire de la sécurité sociale, 1996), 228. On the growth of the mutual society medical infrastructure and the medical profession's response, see also Olivier Faure and Dominique Dessertine, *La maladie entre libéralisme et solidarités, 1850–1940* (Paris: Mutualité Française, 1994), 114–24.

29. Georges Buisson, *Les assurances sociales en danger* (Paris: Edition de la CGT, 1932), 38.

30. Ibid., 39.

31. Code Pénal, book 3, title 2, section 7, paragraph 2, reproduced in Mme de Moro-Giafferi and Dr. Paul Cibrie, *Le secret professionnel médical* (Paris: Mindy, 1934), annexe.

32. Petre Trisca, *Prolégomènes à une déontologie medico-sociale* (Paris: Félix Alcan, 1922), 300.

33. See the prescient remarks of France's minister of public health, Henri Sellier, in a speech at the CSMF's annual meeting in December 1936, *Le Médecin de France* (1 January 1937):, 7–11.

34. Morris Fishbein, "The Doctor and the State," in *The Medical Profession and the Public* (Philadelphia: American Academy of Political and Social Science, 1934), 89, 97.

35. *Journal of the American Medical Association* (hereafter *JAMA*), 3 December 1932, 1952.

36. Rodgers, *Atlantic Crossings,* 429.

37. David Beito, *From Mutual Aid to the Welfare State: Fraternal Societies and Social Services, 1890–1967* (Chapel Hill: University of North Carolina Press, 2000), 219.

38. Franklin Delano Roosevelt, First Inaugural Address, Washington, DC, 4 March 1933.

39. Daniel S. Hirshfield, *The Lost Reform: The Campaign for Compulsory Health Insurance in the United States from 1932 to 1943* (Cambridge, MA: Harvard University Press, 1970), 44–49.

40. Jacob Hacker, *The Divided Welfare State: The Battle over Public and Private Social Benefits in the United States* (Cambridge, U.K.: Cambridge University Press, 2002), 209.

41. Jacob Hacker, "The Historical Logic of National Health Insurance: Structure and Sequence in the Development of British, Canadian, and U.S. Medical Policy," *Studies in American Political Development* 12 (Spring 1998): 57–130, esp. 113.

42. Jill S. Quadagno, "Welfare Capitalism and the Social Security Act of 1935," *American Sociological Review* 49, 5 (October 1984): 632–47, esp. 641.

43. Colin Gordon, *Dead on Arrival: The Politics of Health Care in Twentieth-Century America* (Princeton, NJ: Princeton University Press, 2003), 185.

44. Hirshfield, *The Lost Reform,* 108–30; Klein, *For All These Rights,* 142–43.

45. Morris Fishbein, "Social Aspects of Medical Care," address before the Annual Banquet of the Chicago Hospital Council, 25 January 1939, as quoted by Hirshfield, *The Lost Reform,* 131.

46. Sanford Jacoby, *Modern Manors: Welfare Capitalism since the New Deal* (Princeton, NJ: Princeton University Press, 1997), 5.

47. Beito, *From Mutual Aid to the Welfare State,* 206–15.

48. Robert Cunningham III and Robert M. Cunningham Jr., *The Blues: A History of the Blue Cross and Blue Shield System* (Dekalb: Northern Illinois University Press, 1997), 4.

49. Ibid., 5.

50. Paul Starr, *The Social Transformation of American Medicine,* (New York: Basic Books, 1982), 290.

51. Cunningham and Cunningham, *The Blues,* 6–7.

52. Ibid., 10–22.

53. Starr, *Social Transformation of American Medicine,* 301–303; Rickey Hendricks, *A Model for National Health Care: The History of Kaiser Permanente* (New Brunswick, NJ: Rutgers University Press, 1993), 40, 77–79.

54. *JAMA,* 20 August 1938, 1191–1217.

55. Cunningham and Cunningham, *The Blues*, 44–45, 48–49, 58.

56. Ibid., 15.

57. Klein, *For All These Rights*, 158–59.

58. Cunningham and Cunningham, *The Blues*, 29.

59. Ibid., 76–78, 33, my italics.

60. I borrow the term, though not necessarily the interpretation, from Lawrence D. Brown, "Capture and Culture: Organizational Identity in New York Blue Cross," *Journal of Health Politics, Policy, and Law* 16, 4 (Winter 1991): 658.

4 Challenges and Change during the Second World War, 1940–1945

1. Paul Guérin, *L'Etat contre le* médecin: *Vers une renaissance corporative* (Paris: Editions Médicales Norbert Maloine, 1929), 187.

2. "Les médecins sont-ils satisfaits de leur Ordre?," *Le Figaro*, 30 April 1942.

3. "Code de déontologie et statuts de la profession médicale," *Bulletin de l'Ordre des Médecins* (1941): 12–41.

4. As quoted by Pierre Guillaume, *Rôle du médecin depuis deux siècles, 1800–1945* (Paris: Association pour l'Etude de l'histoire de la sécurité sociale, 1996), 283–84.

5. Miranda Pollard, *Reign of Virtue: Mobilizing Gender in Vichy France* (Chicago: University of Chicago Press, 1998); Francine Muel-Dreyfus, *Vichy et l'éternel féminin: Contribution à une sociologie politique de l'ordre des corps* (Paris: Seuil, 1996); Cheryl A. Koos, "Gender, Anti-individualism, and Nationalism: The Alliance Nationale and the Pronatalist Backlash against the *femme moderne*," *French Historical Studies* 19, 3 (Spring 1996): 699–723.

6. Linda K. Kerber, *Women of the Republic: Intellect and Ideology in Revolutionary America* (Chapel Hill: University of North Carolina Press, 1980); Karen Offen, "Depopulation, Nationalism, and Feminism in Fin-de-Siècle France," *American Historical Review* 89, 3 (1989): 648–76.

7. Remarks of delegate Arnaud, Fédération Nationale de la Mutualité Française, report on the Assemblées, 30 September–2 October 1943, 28–29, 30–31.

8. Louis Portes, *A la Recherche d'une éthique médicale* (Paris, 1954).

9. Chauvet, "Rapport sur les lois sociales de Vichy," 10 May 1942, Archives Nationales de France, box AJ 546.

10. Saul Padover, ed., *The Complete Jefferson* (New York: Irvington Publishers, 1943), 385–86, as quoted by Anatol Lieven, *America Right or Wrong: An Anatomy of American Nationalism* (New York: Oxford University Press, 2004), 30.

11. Jennifer Klein, *For All These Rights, Business, Labor, and the Shaping of America's Public-Private Welfare State* (Princeton, NJ: Princeton University Press, 2003), 166–69.

12. *Journal of the American Medical Association* (hereafter *JAMA*), 13 January 1945, 102.

13. Michael R. Grey, *New Deal Medicine: The Rural Health Programs of the Farm Security Administration* (Baltimore: Johns Hopkins University Press, 1999), 5, 69.

14. Ibid., 4.

15. Ibid., 148–49.

16. Ibid., 30.

17. Morris Fishbein, *History of the American Medical Association* (Philadelphia: Saunders, 1947), 407–8, as quoted by Paul Starr, *The Social Transformation of American Medicine* (New York: Basic Books, 1982), 271.

18. *JAMA*, 13 January 1945, 91–92.

19. Grey, *New Deal Medicine*, 109.

20. Geoffrey Dunn, "Photographic License," *New Times: San Luis Obispo*, 17 January 2002, www.newtimes-slo.com/archives/cov_stories_2002/cov_01172002.html; James Noble Gregory, *American Exodus: The Dust Bowl Migration and Okie Culture in California* (New York: Oxford University Press, 1989), 12–13.

21. *JAMA*, 26 June 1943, 609–11.

22. Grey, *New Deal Medicine*, 156.

23. Alan Derickson, "Health Security for All? Social Unionism and Universal Health Insurance, 1935–1958," *Journal of American History* 80 (March 1994): 1333–56.

24. Klein, *For All These Rights*, 169–72.

25. *JAMA*, 13 January 1945, 103.

26. Klein, *For All These Rights*, 178–80, 182.

27. Alan Derickson, "Health Security for All?" 1333–56, esp. 1352.

28. Jacob Hacker, *The Divided Welfare State: The Battle over Public and Private Social Benefits in the United States* (Cambridge, U.K.: Cambridge University Press, 2002), 214; Derickson, "Health Security for All?" 1333–56, esp. 1351.

5 Labor's Quest for Health Security, 1945–1960

1. "The President's Page," *Journal of the American Medical Association* (hereafter *JAMA*), 24 February 1951 567; 15 January 1949, 156; 19 February 1949, 530–31; Alan Derickson, *Health Security for All: Dreams of Universal Health Care in America* (Baltimore: Johns Hopkins University Press, 2005), 105–10; Jill Quadagno, *One Nation Uninsured: Why the U.S. Has No National Health Insurance* (New York: Oxford University Press), 30–34; Jacob Hacker, *The Divided Welfare State: The Battle over Public and Private Social Benefits in the United States* (Cambridge, U.K.: Cambridge University Press, 2002), 223–25.

2. After Laroque was expelled from the Vichy government in October 1940, an old friend gave him a job in the Lyons silk industry. In December 1942 he was persuaded by Resistance leaders Jean Moulin and Alexandre Parodi to join efforts under way in London. See Laroque, *Au service de l'homme et du droit* (Paris: Association pour l'Etude de l'Histoire de la Sécurité Sociale, 1993), 127–31.

3. Archives Nationales de France (hereafter AN), box 72 AJ 546; also see Andrew Shennan, *Rethinking France: Plans for Renewal 1940–1946* (Oxford, U.K.: Clarendon, 1989).

4. "Salaire minimum et salaire feminin," 18 June 1943, Section sociale, AN, box 72 AJ 546.

5. Antoine Prost, "L'évolution de la politique familiale en France de 1938 à 1981," *Le Mouvement Social* 129 (October–December 1984): 8–12.

6. Author's interview with Pierre Laroque, Paris, 5 December 1995.

7. Bruno Valat, *Histoire de la Sécurité Sociale: 1945–1967, l'État, l'institution et la santé* (Paris: Economica 2001), 30.

8. "L'opinion anglaise devant le Plan Beveridge," January 1943, Section sociale, AN, box 72 AJ 546.

9. "Rapport du Lieutenant Loubere," 3 December 1942, Section sociale, Secrétariat des Commissions, AN, box 72 AJ 546.

10. "Rapport sur l'Etat d'esprit en France au regard d'une forme de gouvernement pour l'après guerre," Direction Générale des Services Spéciaux, Algiers, 23 February 1944, AN, F22 2059. Also see Michel Debré (pseud. Jacquier), *Refaire la France: L'éffort d'une génération* (Paris: Plon, 1945); and Peter Hall, *Governing the Economy: The Politics of State Intervention in Britain and France* (Oxford, U.K.: Oxford University Press, 1986), 140–41.

11. "Rapport de P. Chauvet," n.d., Section sociale, AN, box 72 AJ 546.

12. Laroque, *Au service de l'homme et du droit*, 210–14.

13. "Rapport sur les principaux mesures sociaux à prendre dès la libération, rapporteur: Albert Gazier," January 1944, Commission des Affaires économiques et sociales, Comité sur les problèmes sociaux de la France libérée, AN, box F22 2050. On Michelin, see John F. Sweets, *Choices in Vichy France: The French under German Occupation* (New York: Oxford University Press), 194.

14. Text of a poster of the Fédération Nationale de la Mutualité Française, reprinted in Romain Laveille, *Histoire de la mutualité* (Paris: Hachette, 1964), 163–64.

15. Henry C. Galant, *Histoire politique de la sécurité sociale française, 1945–1952* (Paris: Armand Colin, 1955), 33–34.

16. Laroque, *Au service de l'homme et du droit*, 215.

17. The Christian Democratic CFTC won the majority on seven boards while only two went to independent or mutual coalitions; six boards were evenly split. Galant, *Histoire politique de la sécurité sociale,* 126.

18. Minutes of 25 June 1945, Centre des Archives Contemporaines (hereafter CAC), dossier 1976 0231/17, Conseil Supérieur des Assurances Sociales; *Le Médecin de France,* 20 July 1945.

19. Ordonnance no. 45-2454, 19 October 1945, *Journal Officiel de la République Française*. See esp. articles 10, 12, and 13.

20. J. Rodgers Hollingsworth, Jerald Hage, and Robert A. Hanneman, *State Intervention in Medical Care: Consequences for Britain, France, Sweden, and the United States, 1890–1970* (Ithaca, NY: Cornell University Press, 1990), chaps. 3 and 4.

21. Preamble of the constitution of the World Health Organization, 22 July 1946.

22. *Le Concours Médical,* 11 June 1960, 3106.

23. Daniel Fox, *Health Policies, Health Politics: The British and American Experience, 1911–1965* (Princeton, NJ: Princeton University Press, 1986), 152; *Bulletin de la Confédération Nationale du Patronat Français* (hereafter *Bulletin de la CNPF*) 191 (December 1959): 12–19; Jean de Kervasdoué and Jean-François Lacronique, "L'Etat et la technique: L'apparition du rationnement," in *La santé rationnée?* ed. Jean de Kervasdoué, John Kimberly, and Victor Rodwin (Paris: Economica, 1981), 89–115.

24. *Bulletin de la CNPF* 191 (December 1959): 13.

25. Paul Starr, *The Social Transformation of American Medicine* (New York: Basic Books, 1982), 384.

26. Herman M. Somers and Anne R. Somers, *Doctors, Patients, and Health Insurance* (Washington, DC: Brookings Institution, 1967), 199, 176.

27. *Revue de la Sécurité Sociale* 104 (July–August 1959): 62.

28. Fox, *Health Policies, Health Politics,* 169.

29. Raymond Munts, *Bargaining for Health: Labor Unions, Health Insurance, and Medical Care* (Madison: University of Wisconsin Press, 1967), 149.

30. Starr, *Social Transformation of American Medicine,* 385.

31. Minutes of the Conseil d'Administration, Fédération Nationale des Organismes de la Sécurité Sociale, 19 November 1958, CAC dossier 1977 1537/21, 294.

32. Ibid., 9 October 1951, CAC dossier 1977 1537/20.

33. Ibid., 3 February 1947, CAC dossier 1977 1537/5.

34. *Le Médecin de France* 26 (April 1948): 1648.

35. "CSMF-FNOSS Negotiations, 11 February 1952," ibid., 5335–36; "Doctrine Syndicale," ibid., 5370.

36. Letter from Woodrow L. Ginsburg, United Rubber Workers Research Director, to George Guernsey, AFL-CIO Education Department, 8 June 1956, UAW Research Department Archives, Detroit; Bulletin of the San Francisco Medical Society, May 1950, 18; Official Bulletin of the San Francisco Labor Council, 18 November 1953, as quoted by Munts, *Bargaining for Health,* 146–47.

37. *Revue de la Sécurité Sociale* 28 (November 1952): 14–15.

38. Ibid., (October–November 1951): 2–3.

39. Paul V. Dutton, *Origins of the French Welfare State: The Struggle for Social Reform in France* (New York: Cambridge University Press, 2002), 217–18.

40. "Communication sur les problèmes posés par la situation financière du régime général de la Sécurité Sociale" Archives du Comité d'Histoire de la Sécurité Sociale (1950), 17–18.

41. *Le Médecin de France* 75 (May 1952): 5368.

42. Starr, *Social Transformation of American Medicine,* 313.

43. Munts, *Bargaining for Health,* 9, 69; Marie Gottschalk, *The Shadow Welfare State: Labor, Business, and the Politics of Health Care in the United States* (Ithaca, NY: Cornell University Press, 2000), 48.

44. Klein, *For All These Rights,* 224–26.

45. *New York Times,* 19 November 1957, 35, quoted by Gerald Markowitz and David Rosner, "Seeking Common Ground: A History of Labor and Blue Cross," *Journal of Health Politics, Policy, and Law* 16, 4 (Winter 1991): 708.

46. *New York Times,* 27 December 1957, 18; 8 June 1958, E9, quoted by Markowitz and Rosner, "Seeking Common Ground," 709.

47. *New York Times,* 23 May 1959, 50, quoted by Markowitz and Rosner, "Seeking Common Ground," 710–11.

48. As quoted by Robert Cunningham III and Robert M. Cunningham Jr., *The Blues: A History of the Blue Cross and Blue Shield System* (Dekalb: Northern Illinois University Press, 1997), 96n, 272–73.

49. Report of the 3e Congrès Confédéral of the CGT-FO, 12–15 November 1952, 223; report of the 4e Congrès Confédéral of the CGT-FO, 22–25 November 1954, 209; Assemblée Générale, FNOSS, 23–24 May 1956, 63.

50. Ivana Krajcinovic, *From Company Doctors to Managed Care: The United Mine Workers Noble Experiment* (Ithaca, NY: Cornell University Press, 1997); Joseph W. Garbarino, *Health Plans and Collective Bargaining* (Berkeley: University of California Press, 1960), 149–51.

51. Minutes of the Comité Consultatif de la FNOSS, 26 October 1947, CAC dossier 1977 1537/5.

52. Garbarino, *Health Plans and Collective Bargaining,* 158–59.

53. *Le Médecin de France* 108 (February 1955): 8303–5.

54. *Revue de la Mutualité* 10 (June 1958): 4–6.

55. Garbarino, *Health Plans and Collective Bargaining,* 93–97.

56. Munts, *Bargaining for Health,* 61–63.

57. Garbarino, *Health Plans and Collective Bargaining,* chap. 8.

6 The Choice of Public or Private, 1950–1970

1. J. R. Debray, "A propos d'un voyage d'étude effectué aux Etats-Unis, *Bulletin de l'Ordre des Médecins* 4 (December 1951): 280–90.

2. *Journal of the American Medical Association* (hereafter *JAMA*), 17 March 1945, 656.

3. As quoted by Frank D. Campion, *The AMA and U.S. Health Policy since 1940* (Chicago: Chicago Review Press, 1984), 162.

4. *Business Week*, 13 May 1950, quoted by Jennifer Klein, *For All These Rights, Business, Labor, and the Shaping of America's Public-Private Welfare State* (Princeton, NJ: Princeton University Press, 2003), 219.

5. Monte Poen, *Harry Truman versus the Medical Lobby: The Genesis of Medicare* (Columbia: University of Missouri Press), 151.

6. Jean-Daniel Reynaud and Antoinette Catrice-Lorey, *Les assurés et la Sécurité Sociale: Etude sur les assurés du régime général en 1958* (Paris: Comité d'Histoire de la Sécurité Sociale, 1996), 198.

7. *Fortune*, December 1944, 156.

8. Franz Goldman, "Labor's Attitude toward Health Insurance," *Industrial and Labor Relations Review* 2, 1 (October 1948): 90–98.

9. Poen, *Harry Truman versus the Medical Lobby*, 152.

10. Alan Derickson, "Health Security for All? Social Unionism and Universal Health Insurance, 1935–1958," *Journal of American History* 80, 4 (March 1994): 1333–56, esp. 1342–45, 1351; Marie Gottschalk, *The Shadow Welfare State: Labor, Business, and the Politics of Health Care in the United States* (Ithaca, NY: Cornell University Press, 2000), 43; Colin Gordon, *Dead on Arrival: The Politics of Health Care in Twentieth-Century America* (Princeton, NJ: Princeton University Press, 2003), 72–82.

11. Quoted by Edwin Witte, "Organized Labor and Social Security," in *Labor and the New Deal*, ed. Milton Derber and Edwin Young (Madison: University of Wisconsin Press, 1957), 271.

12. Gordon, *Dead on Arrival*, 231–32.

13. Jacob Hacker, *The Divided Welfare State: The Battle over Public and Private Social Benefits in the United States* (Cambridge, U.K.: Cambridge University Press, 2002), 243.

14. Michael K. Brown, "Bargaining for Social Rights: Unions and the Reemergence of Welfare Capitalism," *Political Science Quarterly* 112, 4 (Winter 1997–1998): 645–74, esp. 665. "Union shops" remained legal but cumbersome, and the Taft-Hartley Act explicitly recognized state labor laws that restricted their creation. For more on this, see ibid., 663–64.

15. Gottschalk, *Shadow Welfare State*, 46.

16. Robert Cunningham III and Robert M. Cunningham Jr., *The Blues: A History of the Blue Cross and Blue Shield System* (Dekalb: Northern Illinois University Press, 1997), 100; Raymond Munts, *Bargaining for Health: Labor Unions, Health Insurance, and Medical Care* (Madison: University of Wisconsin Press, 1967), 136.

17. Uwe E. Reinhardt, "How the Devil Subverted the Nation's Soul: An Allegory About American Health Policy," *Proceedings of the Third Conference of the National Academy of Social Insurance* (Dubuque, IA: Kendall/Hunt, 1992), 75–93.

18. Senator Taft et al., "Federal Labor Relations Act of 1947," supplemental views, 52, quoted by Gottschalk, *Shadow Welfare State*, 47.

19. Klein, "Bargaining for Social Rights," 230–31.

20. "Blueprint of Proposed Industry Program," October 1956, Orville Grahame papers, University of Iowa Special Collections, box 18, quoted Gordon, *Dead on Arrival*, 192–93.

21. Hacker, *Divided Welfare State*, 239–43.

22. See chap. 3.

23. Letter from Prime Minister Michel Debré to Dr. Monier, 14 April 1962, Centre des Archives Contemporaines (hereafter CAC), dossier 1976 0235/4; *Revue de la Sécurité Sociale* 115 (July–August 1960): 44–47.

24. Report of the Conseil d'Administration, Confédération des Syndicats Médicaux Français (hereafter CSMF), 19–21 February 1960; *Le Médecin de France* 170 (April 1960): 372–73.

25. *JAMA*, 30 June 1951, 826–27. Since 1940, the International Brotherhood of Teamsters has been the single largest private sector union in the United States. Beck became IBT president shortly after his appearance at the AMA dinner; he was sent to prison for larceny and tax evasion in 1958.

26. Letter from Charles Veillon to Doctor Valingot, 27 June 1960, CAC dossier 1977 1537/68.

27. Report of the Conseil d'Administration, CSMF, 19–21 February 1960; *Le Médecin de France* 170 (April 1960): 373.

28. Minutes of the Tenth General Assembly of the Conseil National du Patronat Français (CNPF), *Bulletin du CNPF*, 5 February 1951, 4.

29. André Brossard, report of the Chambre de Commerce de Paris, *Revue Française du Travail* (March–April 1949): 185. Brossard's report was later adopted as the official position of the Assembly of Presidents of the Chambers of Commerce. See also the response to the Brossard report by Minister of Labor Samson, 187–95.

30. Letter from Georges Villiers, president of the CNPF, to presidents of all member associations, 14 March 1957, *Bulletin du CNPF* 159 (April 1957): 7.

31. *Le Monde*, 25 March 1960.

32. *Le Concours Médical*, 24 September 1960, 4236; memorandum from Minister of Labor Paul Bacon to Prime Minister Michel Debré, 13 October 1959, 6, CAC dossier 1976 0235/3.

33. *La Médecine Humaine et Sociale* 1 (December 1961): 3–8; (January 1962): 3–5.

34. Bruno Valat, *Histoire de la Sécurité Sociale: 1945–1967, l'État, l'institution et la santé* (Paris: Economica 2001), 417, 443; *Le Médecin de France* (February 1964): 849.

35. *Le Médecin de France* 203 (January 1963): 24.

36. *Le Médecin de France* 213 (December 1963): 691–92.

37. *Revue de la Sécurité Sociale* 172 (November 1965): 4.

38. Anne R. Somers and Herman M. Somers, "Health Insurance: Are Cost and Quality Controls Necessary?" *Industrial and Labor Relations Review* 13, 4 (July 1960): 581; *JAMA*, 31 March 1962, 17.

39. On Gompers's opposition to compulsory health insurance, see chap. 2; *JAMA*, 12 August 1961, 21–22.

40. Minutes of the Twenty-first General Assembly of the CNPF, *Bulletin du CNPF*, 10 July 1956, 110; Cathie Jo Martin, "Together Again: Business, the Government and the Quest for Cost Control," *Journal of Health Politics, Policy, and Law* 18, 2 (1993): 369, quoted by Jill Quadagno, *One Nation Uninsured: Why the U.S. Has No Health Insurance* (New York: Oxford University Press, 2005), 121.

41. *JAMA*, 4 January 1965, 135.

42. *Le Monde*, 25 March 1960; *JAMA*, 12 August 1961, 368–69; 19 August 1961, 22.

43. Ibid.

44. Gordon, *Dead on Arrival*, 238.

45. *Le Médecin de France* 176 (October 1960): 913; Johnson, quoted by Robert Dallek, *Flawed Giant: Lyndon Johnson and His Times* (New York: Oxford University Press, 1998), 209–10.

46. "Health Areas for Discussion," 22 September 1965, Wilbur Cohen papers, State Historical Society of Wisconsin, box 120:3, as quoted by Gordon, *Dead on Arrival*, 239; *JAMA*, 24 May 1965, 15.

47. *JAMA,* 12 August 1961, 21; confidential report of the ALC-HIAA-LIAA Task Force, 8 January 1965, Orville Grahame paper, University of Iowa, box 25, quoted by Gordon, *Dead on Arrival,* 237.

48. Hacker, *Divided Welfare State,* 245.

49. Gordon, *Dead on Arrival,* 235.

50. For a comprehensive account of Medicaid, see Robert Stevens and Rosemary Stevens, *Welfare Medicine in America: A Case Study of Medicaid* (New Brunswick, NJ: Transaction, 2003).

51. Theodore Marmor, *The Politics of Medicare,* 2nd ed. (Hawthorne, NY: Aldine de Gruyter, 2000), chap. 4.

52. Wilbur Cohen, "Random Reflections on the Great Society's Politics and Health Care Programs after Twenty Years," in *The Great Society and Its Legacy: Twenty Years of U.S. Social Policy,* ed. Marshal Kaplan and Peggy Cuciti (Durham, NC: Duke University Press, 1986), 118; Cunningham and Cunningham, *The Blues,* 151.

53. Paul Starr, *The Social Transformation of American Medicine* (New York: Basic Books, 1982), 375.

54. United States Commission on Civil Rights, *The Federal Civil Rights Enforcement Effort—One Year Later* (1971), 11, 130, quoted by Gordon, *Dead on Arrival,* 202.

55. Marmor, *Politics of Medicare,* 53.

56. Adapted from Jean Bernard, *Discours au Congrès international de morale médicale* (1966), cited by David Wilsford, *Doctors and the State: The Politics of Health Care in France and the United States* (Durham, NC: Duke University Press, 1991), 1.

57. Deborah Chollet, "Employment-Based Health Insurance in a Changing Work Force, *Health Affairs* 13, 1 (1994): 315–21.

58. Valat, *Histoire de la Sécurité Sociale,* 496.

7 Cost Control Moves to the Fore, 1970–2000

1. Marie-Thérèse Join-Lambert et al., *Politiques sociales* (Paris: Fondation Nationale des Sciences Politiques et Dalloz, 1994), 47–67.

2. Quoted by Robert Cunningham III and Robert M. Cunningham Jr., *The Blues: A History of the Blue Cross and Blue Shield System* (Dekalb: Northern Illinois University Press, 1997), 168.

3. Quoted by Bernard Gibaud, *Clément Michel, la passion de la solidarité* (Paris: Association pour l'Etude de l'Histoire de la Sécurité Sociale, 1993), 52.

4. David Wilsford, *Doctors and the State: The Politics of Health Care in France and the United States* (Durham, NC: Duke University Press, 1991), 10–14; Jean de Kervasdoué and Victor Rodwin, "La politique de santé et le rôle de l'Etat, 1945–1980," in *La Santé rationnée?* ed. Jean de Kervasdoué, John Kimberly, and Victor Rodwin (Paris: Economica, 1981), 29.

5. Computed Tomography (CT) and Magnetic Resonance Imaging (MRI) are noninvasive methods to view the internal workings of the body, permitting faster and more accurate diagnoses than previously possible.

6. Diana B. Dutton, *Worse than the Disease: Pitfalls of Medical Progress* (Cambridge, U.K.: Cambridge University Press, 1987); Wilsford, *Doctors and the State,* 15–18.

7. Jean de Kervasdoué, *Santé: Pour une révolution sans réforme* (Paris: Gallimard 1999), 17.

8. Wilsford, *Doctors and the State,* 17.

9. Frank A. Sloan, "Arrow's Concept of the Health Care Consumer: A Forty-Year Retrospective," *Journal of Health Politics, Policy and Law* 26, 5 (October 2001): 899–911; Colin Gordon, *Dead on Arrival: The Politics of Health Care in Twentieth-Century America* (Princeton, NJ: Princeton University Press, 2003), 158–59.

10. *Le Concours Médical,* 28 November 1970, 2053–60.

11. Vivien Schmidt, *From State to Market: The Transformation of French Business and Government* (Cambridge, U.K.: Cambridge University Press, 1996), 73–76.

12. Peter Hall, *Governing the Economy: The Politics of State Intervention in Britain and France* (New York: Oxford University Press, 1986), 140, 162–63.

13. *Le Médecin de France* 288 (April 1970): 24; 290 (July–August 1970): 26–28.

14. Michel Lucas, "La Convention nationale entre la Sécurité sociale et le corps medical," *Droit Social,* nos. 9–10 (1971): 585.

15. *Le Médecin de France,* 287 (March 1970), 32–36.

16. François Steudler, "Médecine libérale et conventionnement," *Sociologie du Travail* 2, 77 (April–June 1977): 176–98.

17. *Le Médecin de France* 292 (October 1970): 27.

18. Ibid. 285 (January 1970): 4.

19. Ibid. 294 (December 1970): 34–35.

20. Ibid., p. 32.

21. Ibid. 294 (December 1970): 18–35.

22. Steudler, "Médecine libérale et conventionnement," 194n.

23. Douglas Coleman, "An Analysis of the Components of Rising Costs," in the HEW's *Report on the National Conference on Medical Costs,* 95, as quoted by Cunningham and Cunningham, *The Blues,* p. 165.

24. Senate Labor Committee, *Health Care Crisis* (1971), 883, as quoted by Cunningham and Cunningham, *The Blues,* 279n. 20.

25. Pierre de Vise, "The Sixty-Year Debate over National Health Insurance," Brief submitted to U.S. Congress House Ways and Means Committee, 1970, 37, quoted by Cunningham and Cunningham, *The Blues,* 186.

26. W. R. Grace executive quoted by Gordon, *Dead on Arrival,* 244.

27. For more on Kaiser, see chaps. 4–6 and Rickey Hendricks, *A Model for National Health Care: The History of Kaiser-Permanente* (New Brunswick, NJ: Rutgers University Press, 1993).

28. Paul Starr, *The Social Transformation of American Medicine* (New York: Basic Books, 1982), 395–96.

29. Transcript of Oval Office Conversation 450-23, 17 February 1971, 5:26 PM–5:53 PM, http://whitehousetapes.org/.

30. Paul Starr, *Social Transformation,* 396. See also Theodore R. Marmor, *The Politics of Medicare,* 2nd ed. (New York: Aldine de Gruyter, 2000), 102.

31. Cunningham and Cunningham, *The Blues,* 183.

32. Jennifer Klein, *For All These Rights, Business, Labor, and the Shaping of America's Public-Private Welfare State* (Princeton, NJ: Princeton University Press, 2003), 269; Lawrence Brown, *Politics and Health Care Organization: HMOs as Federal Policy* (Washington, DC: Brookings Institution, 1983), 265–70.

33. Rashi Fein, *Medical Care, Medical Costs: The Search for Health Insurance Policy* (Cambridge, MA: Harvard University Press, 1986), 137; Burton Beam and John McFadden, *Employee Benefits,* 6th ed. (Chicago: Dearborn, 2004), 194.

34. Jean de Kervasdoué, ed., *Le carnet de santé de la France en 2000* (Paris: Mutualité Française, 2000), 76.

35. "The New Federalism in Health: Shifting Responsibilities and Reducing Costs into the 80s," *Journal of the American Medical Association* (hereafter *JAMA*), 4 June 1982, 2911–12.

36. Quoted by Jacob Hacker, *The Divided Welfare State: The Battle over Public and Private Social Benefits in the United States* (Cambridge, U.K.: Cambridge University Press, 2002), 259.

37. *Le Médecin de France*, 10 June 1980, 6. Five percent of those queried did not select any of the responses provided. *Le Médecin de France*, 29 April 1980, 6; Renée Hélène Bellon, "Le syndicalisme médical libéral," 101–103.

38. *Le Médecin de France*, 29 April 1980, 7.

39. Bellon, "Le syndicalisme médical," 101.

40. Paul Godt, "Health Care: The Political Economy of Social Policy," in *Policy-Making in France*, ed. Paul Godt (London: Pinter, 1989), 191–207, esp. 200.

41. Wilsford, *Doctors and the State,* 111.

42. *JAMA,* 7 September 1984), 1133.

43. Fein, *Medical Care, Medical Costs,* 71.

44. *JAMA,* 9 December 1983, 3039.

45. James C. Robinson, "The Dynamics and Limits of Corporate Growth in Health Care," *Health Affairs* 15, 2 (Summer 1996): 155–69; John K. Iglehart, "The Struggle between Managed Care and Fee-for-Service Practice," *New England Journal of Medicine,* 7 July 1994, 63–67.

46. David Wilsford, "The State and the Medical Profession in France," in *The Changing Medical Profession,* ed. Frederic W. Hafferty and John B. McKinlay (New York: Oxford, 1993), 124–37.

47. Victor G. Rodwin, "The Rise of Managed Care in the United States: Lessons for French Health Policy," in *Health Policy Reform, National Schemes and Globalization,* ed. C. Altenstetter and J. Björkman (New York: St. Martin's, 1997), 41–47; Claude Béraud, "Les transformations du système de soins au cours des 20 dernières années: Point de vue d'un acteur," *Sciences Sociales et Santé* 20, 4: 35–74.

48. Morris Fishbein, "The Doctor and the State," *The Medical Profession and the Public: Papers from the Meeting of the American Academy of Political and Social Science*" (Philadelphia: The American Academy of Political and Social Science, 1934), 97.

49. *JAMA,* 19 November 1982, 2457–58.

50. *JAMA,* 25 November 1983, 2773.

51. Benjamin G. Druss et al., "Chronic Illness and Plan Satisfaction under Managed Care," *Health Affairs* 19, 1 (January/February 2000): 203–9.

52. Marc A. Rodwin, "Physicians' Conflicts of Interest in HMOs and Hospitals," in *Conflicts Of Interest in Clinical Practice and Research,* ed. Roy Spece Jr., David Shimm, and Allen Buchanan (New York: Oxford University Press, 1995), 208. See also Marc A. Rodwin, *Medicine, Money, and Morals: Physicians' Conflicts of Interest* (New York: Oxford University Press, 1995).

53. Rodwin, "Physicians' Conflicts of Interest," 208.

54. David Dranove, *The Economic Evolution of American Health Care: From Marcus Welby to Managed Care* (Princeton, NJ: Princeton University Press, 2000), 87, 85–86.

55. Dana E. Johnson, "Life, Death, and the Dollar Sign: Medical Ethics and the Cost Containment," *JAMA,* 13 July 1984, 224. For a longer view, see David Mechanic, "Managed Care and the Imperative For a New Professional Ethic," *Health Affairs* 19, 5 (September–October 2000): 100–111.

56. Frank J. Jirka Jr., "Three Major Challenges: Quality, Cost, and Balance," *JAMA,* 13 April 1984, 1867–68.

57. Helen Darling, "Employers and Managed Care: What Are the Early Returns," *Health Affairs* (Winter 1991): 147–60.

58. Quoted in Iglehart, "The Struggle between Managed Care and Fee-for-Service Practice," 66.

59. Ibid.

8 Hospitals and the Difficult Art of Health Care Reform, 1980–Present

1. Clément Michel, "L'hôpital et la *Sécurité Sociale*," *Techniques hospitalières* no. 109 (June 1954): 45, quoted by Bruno Valat, *Histoire de la Sécurité Sociale: 1945–1967, l'Etat, l'institution et la santé* (Paris: Economica 2001), 203–4.

2. Gérard de Pouvourville, "Differences in the Approaches of the Doctor, Manager, Politician and Social Scientist in Health Care Controversies—Hospital Case-Mix Management Methods," *Social Science and Medicine* 29, 3 (1989): 341–49, 345; Marie-Thérèse Join-Lambert et al., *Politiques sociales* (Paris: Fondation Nationale des Sciences Politiques et Dalloz, 1994), 394–98.

3. "OECD in Figures: Statistics on Member Countries," *OECD Observer* (2005), Supplement 1, 8.

4. Paul Starr, *The Social Transformation of American Medicine* (New York: Basic Books, 1982), 349–51.

5. De Pouvourville, "Differences in the Approaches," 341–49.

6. Jean-Marie Rodrigues and Béatrice Trombert-Paviot, "Case Mix in France: Is There a French Way from the Problem to Paradigm in Healthcare? The DRG/PMSI Saga," in *Case Mix: Global Views, Local Actions*, ed. F. H. Roger France et al. (Washington, DC: IOS Press, 2001), 57–66.

7. Rashi Fein, *Medical Care, Medical Costs: The Search for Health Insurance Policy* (Cambridge, MA: Harvard University Press, 1986), 86–87.

8. Theodore R. Marmor, *The Politics of Medicare*, 2nd ed. (New York: Aldine de Gruyter, 2000), 110–13.

9. Robert Cunningham III and Robert M. Cunningham Jr., *The Blues: A History of the Blue Cross and Blue Shield System* (Dekalb: Northern Illinois University Press, 1997), 208.

10. Rodrigues and Trombert-Paviot, "Case Mix in France," 58.

11. Béatrice Majnoni d'Intignano, *Economie de la Santé* (Paris: Presses Universitaires de France, 2001), 346–49.

12. De Pouvourville, "Differences in the Approaches," 345–46.

13. Uwe Reinhardt, "Spending More through 'Cost Control': Our Obsessive Quest to Gut the Hospital," *Health Affairs* 15 (Summer 1996): 145–54, esp. 146–47.

14. Rosanna M. Coffey and Daniel Z. Louis, "Case Mix in the USA: Fifteen Years of DRG-Based Financing in the United States," in France et al., *Case Mix,* 159–72, esp. 164.

15. Reinhardt, "Spending More through 'Cost Controls,'" 146.

16. *New York Times*, 29 June 1995, B1, as quoted by Reinhardt, "Spending More through 'Cost Controls,'" 146.

17. Béatrice Majnoni d'Intignano, "Politique de la santé Médecine libérale: Le débat confisqué," *Le Monde*, 24 February 1990.

18. "Un entretien avec M. René Teulade," *Le Monde*, 14 October 1992.

19. Because of an absence of specific French census data, it is difficult to know the life expectancy of disadvantaged minorities in France. Nor can we be sure exactly how Teulade

defined "outside the health care system." When he made the remark, it had been a long time since a third of Americans were without health coverage of any kind.

20. "Assurance maladie: Ce qui bloque la réforme: Conservatisme ou gestion d'amateurs?" interview with Béatrice Majnoni d'Intignano by Agnès Verdier, *Société Civile* no. 32 (January 2004), www.ifrap.org/Sante/Entretien-BMI.htm; Victor R. Fuchs, "The Best Health Care System in the World?" *JAMA,* 19 August 1992, 916–17.

21. Raymond Soubie, et al., *Santé 2010: Equité et efficacité du système* (Paris: Documentation Française, 1993), see preface and 29, 143–72.

22. Caisse Nationale d'Assurance Maladie des Travailleurs Salariés (CNAMTS), "Démographie médicale," *Le Médecin de France,* 29 April–6 May 1993, 5–10.

23. Jean-Michel Normand, "Conflits de générations et divorce entre deux conceptions de la médecine libérale," *Le Monde,* 19 January 1990; *Le Médecin de France,* 29 April–6 May 1993, 8–12.

24. Jean-Michel Normand, "Conflits de générations."

25. Marie C. Reed and Paul B. Ginsburg, "Behind the Times: Physician Income, 1995–1999," *Data Bulletin 24* (March 2003).

26. Jacob Hacker, *The Divided Welfare State: The Battle over Public and Private Social Benefits in the United States* (Cambridge, U.K.: Cambridge University Press, 2002), 264.

27. Richard A. Wright, "Community Oriented Primary Care: The Cornerstone of Health Care Reform," *JAMA,* 19 May 1993, 2544–47, esp. 2545.

28. Lawrence O. Gostin and Alan I. Widiss, "What's Wrong with the ERISA Vacuum?" *JAMA,* 19 May 1993, 2527–32, esp. 2528.

29. *Curtiss Wright Corp. v. Schoonejongen et al.* 514 U.S. 73, 78 (1995). See Rand E. Rosenblatt, Testimony before the Subcommittee on Employer-Employee Relations of the Committee on Education and the Workforce of the United States House of Representatives, hearing on "ERISA: A Quarter Century of Providing Workers Health Insurance," 24 February 1999, www.house.gov/ed_workforce/hearings/106th/eer/erisa22499/rosenblatt.htm.

30. Cunningham and Cunningham, *The Blues,* 218; Marie Gottschalk, *The Shadow Welfare State, Labor, Business, and the Politics of Health Care in the United States* (Ithaca, NY: Cornell University Press, 2000), 53–57.

31. Gostin and Widiss, "What's Wrong with the ERISA Vacuum"? 2528.

32. Rosenblatt, Testimony before the Subcommittee on Employer-Employee Relations.

33. As cited by Theda Skocpol, *Boomerang: Health Care Reform and the Turn against Government* (New York: Norton, 1997), 27. Skocpol provides an excellent and accessible analysis of how the Clinton team conceived health care reform, their triumphs and their missteps.

34. Ibid., 28, 37.

35. President William Jefferson Clinton, *State of the Union Address,* 25 January 1994.

36. Robert Skidelsky, *John Maynard Keynes: The Economist as Savior, 1920–1937* (New York: Penguin, 1992), xxii–xxiii.

37. Gottschalk, *Shadow Welfare State,* 137–43.

38. Marmor, *Politics of Medicare,* 133.

39. Skocpol, *Boomerang,* chap. 2.

40. Gottschalk, *Shadow Welfare State,* 146.

41. Mike Lux, "Interest Group Positioning," memo to President Clinton, 15 December 1993, 1, quoted by Skocpol, *Boomerang,* 96.

42. Carolyn Pemberton and Deborah Holmes, eds., *EBRI Databook on Employee Benefits,* 3rd ed. (Washington, DC: EBRI, 1995), 261, as cited by Gottschalk, *Shadow Welfare State,* 123.

43. See chap. 7.

44. Robert J. Blendon et al., "Making the Critical Choices," *JAMA*, 13 May 1992, 2509–20, esp. 2516; George D. Lundberg, "American Health Care System Management Objectives: The Aura of Inevitability Becomes Incarnate," *JAMA*, 19 May 1993, 2555.

45. As quoted by Robert Pear, "Health Care Tug-of-War Puts AMA under Strain," *New York Times*, 5 August 1994.

46. Skocpol, *Boomerang*, 171–72.

47. Gottschalk, *Shadow Welfare State*, 155.

48. *Le Monde*, 6 September 1995.

49. Philippe C. Schmitter, "Still the Century of Corporatism?" in *Trends Towards Corporatist Intermediation*, ed. Philippe C. Schmitter and Gerhard Lehmbruch (London: Sage, 1979), 7–48.

50. Skocpol, *Boomerang*, 55–60.

51. William Saffran, *The French Polity*, 4th ed. (White Plains, NY: Longman, 1995), 152–55.

52. Edouard Balladur, "Lettre de mission," 24 March 1994, Raymond Soubie, Jean-Louis Portos, Christian Prieur, *Livre blanc sur le système de santé et d'assurance maladie* (Paris: La Documentation Française, 1994), 10.

53. Ibid., 183, 185.

54. Ibid., 228.

55. Ibid., 213–15.

56. *Le Point*, 2 September 1995.

57. Alain Juppé, "Déclaration de politique générale sur la réforme de la protection sociale à l'Assemblée Nationale, 15 novembre 1995," *Le Monde*, 17 November 1997.

58. See chap. 5.

59. "La Contribution Sociale Généralisée," Quatorzième rapport au Président de la République (analyse), 14 June 2005.

60. Majnoni d'Intignano, *Économie de la santé*, 28.

61. "La Contribution Sociale Généralisée."

62. See esp. the remarks of large employers and union leaders in *Livre blanc*, 395, 443.

63. Gilles Johanet, *Santé: Dépenser sans compter, des pensées sans conter* (Paris: Santé de France, 1994), 7; Jean-Pierre Dumont, *Les systèmes de protection sociale en Europe* (Paris: Economica, 1995), 19, 75–77, 89–95; "La répartition des interventions entre les assurances maladies obligatoires et complémentaires en matière de dépenses de santé," Commission des Comptes de la Sécurité Sociale, directed by Jean-François Chadelat (Paris: La Documentation Française, 2003), 10–11; Commissariat Général du Plan, *Santé 2010* 253, 257–58.

64. Soubie et al., *Santé 2010*, 137–40.

65. Thomas C. Buchmueller and Agnes Couffinhal, "Private Health Insurance in France," *OECD Working Papers 12* 3 (March 2004): 13–15; A, Bocognano et al., "La complémentaire maladie en France: Qui bénéficie de quels remboursements? Résultats de l'enquête Santé Protection Sociale 1998," *Questions d'économie de la santé* 32 (October 2000): 1–6.

66. Juppé, "Déclaration de politique générale."

67. Majnoni d'Intignano, *Economie de la santé*, 313

68. Juppé, "Déclaration de politique générale."

69. Claude Maffioli, "La place du practicien dans la maîtrise des dépenses de santé," in *La maîtrise des dépenses de santé en Europe et en Amérique du Nord,* ed. Etienne Douat (Rennes: Université de Rennes, 1996), 254–58.

70. Juppé, "Déclaration de politique générale."

71. Christian Saint-Etienne, *L'Etat mensonger* (Paris: Editions JC Lattès, 1996), 80, as quoted by Timothy Smith, *France in Crisis: Welfare, Inequality and Globalization since 1980* (Cambridge, U.K.: Cambridge University Press, 2004), 145.

72. Juppé, "Déclaration de politique générale."

73. "Les professions de santé embarrassés par la réforme de la protection sociale," *Le Monde*, 29 November 1995.

74. "Médecins: Trois organisations appellent une journée d'action," *Le Monde*, 3 December 1995.

75. "Les professions de santé embarrassés par la réforme de la protection sociale," *Le Monde*, 29 November 1995; "Les médecins défilent contre 'le rationnement des soins,'" *Le Monde*, 17 December 1995.

76. "Les professions de santé embarrassés par la réforme de la protection sociale," *Le Monde*, 29 November 1995.

77. "Le premier ministre calme les médecins," *Le Monde*, 19 January 1996.

78. Béatrice Majnoni D'Intignano, "Réformer sans conflit? L'exemple de la médecine," *Commentaire* 25, 97 (Spring 2002): 41.

79. Study of the Services de Statistiques, Ministère du Travail et des Affaires Sociales, cited by *Le Monde*, 7 January 1996.

80. Gilles Johanet, quoted by *Le Monde*, 7 January 1996.

81. David M. Walker, "Health Care System Crisis: Growing Challenges Point to Need for Fundamental Reform" (Washington, DC: General Accounting Office, 2004), 22.

82. Milt Freudenheim, "Using New Medicare Billions, HMOs Again Court Elderly," *New York Times*, 9 March 2004; Robert A. Berenson, "Medicare Disadvantaged and the Search for the Elusive 'Level Playing Field,'" *Health Affairs*, 15 December 2004, Web exclusive, DOI: 10.1377/hlthaff.w4.572.

83. *Economic Report of the President Transmitted to the Congress* (Washington, DC: U.S. Government Printing Office, 2005), 130.

84. Transcript of the president's speech from "Health Care Coverage Debate," *The Online NewsHour*, PBS, 16 February 2006, www.pbs.org/newshour/bb/health/jan-june06/coverage_2-16.html.

85. Karen Davis et al., "How High Is Too High? Implications of High-Deductible Health Plans," *The Commonwealth Fund*, 1–3, www.cmwf.org/publications/publications_show.htm?doc_id=274007.

86. Arnold S. Relman, "The Health of Nations: Medicine and the Free Market," *New Republic*, 7 March 2005, 23–30.

87. Jonathan Gruber, "The Cost and Coverage Impact of the President's Health Insurance Budget Proposals," Center on Budget and Policy Priorities, 15 February 2006, www.cbpp.org/2-15-06health.htm.

9 Les Jeux Sont Faits? 2000–Present

1. John Sheils and Randall Haught, "The Cost of Tax-Exempt Health Benefits in 2004," *Health Affairs*, 25 February 2004, DOI: 10.1377/hlthaff.W4.106; Todd Gilmer and Richard Kronick, "It's the Premiums, Stupid: Projections of the Uninsured through 2013," *Health Affairs*, 5 April 2005, Web exclusive, DOI 10.1377hlthaff.W5.143.

2. For an excellent summary of the limited potential of consumer price shopping in health care, see Paul B. Ginsburg, "Testimony before the U.S. House of Representatives, Committee on Energy and Commerce, Subcommittee on Health," 15 March 2006, Center for Studying Health System Change, http://www.hschange.com/CONTENT/823/; Deborah

Stone, "How Market Ideology Guarantees Racial Inequality," in *Healthy, Wealthy, and Fair: Health Care and the Good Society,* ed. James A. Morone and Lawrence Jacobs (New York: Oxford University Press, 2005), 65–89.

3. Paul V. Dutton and Bruno Valat, "La réforme de l'assurance maladie aux Etats-Unis et en France (1993–2004)," *Histoire et Sociétés: Revue Européenne d'Histoire Sociale* 11 (July 2004): 49–63; P. Hassenteufel and S. Hennion-Moreau, eds., *Concurrence et protection sociale en Europe* (Rennes: Presses Universitaires de Rennes, 2004).

4. Victor G. Rodwin, "Health Care Reform in France—The Birth of State-Led Managed Care," *New England Journal of Medicine,* 25 November 2004, 2259–62.

5. Geoff Meads et al., *The Case for Interprofessional Collaboration in Health and Social Care* (London: Blackwell, 2005); Suzanne Gordon, *Nursing against the Odds: How Health Care Cost Cutting, Media Stereotypes, And Medical Hubris Undermine Nurses And Patient Care* (Ithaca, NY: Cornell University Press, 2005); Celia Davies, "Getting Health Professionals to Work Together," *British Medical Journal,* 15 April 2000, 1021–22.

6. For more on promising alternative models of care, see David Himmelstein and Steffie Woolhandler, *Bleeding the Patient: The Consequences of Corporate Healthcare* (Monroe, ME: Common Courage Press, 2001); and David Mechanic, *The Truth about Health Care: Why Reform Is Not Working in America* (New Brunswick, NJ: Rutgers University Press, 2006).

7. I borrow the term "silos of solidarity" from Colin Gordon, who adapted it from Joel Rogers. See Colin Gordon, *Dead on Arrival: The Politics of Health Care in Twentieth-Century America* (Princeton, NJ: Princeton University Press, 2003), 282; Joel Rogers, "Divide and Conquer: Further Reflections on the Character of American Labor Laws," *Wisconsin Law Review* 1 (1990): 1–147. Also see Marie Gottschalk, "Organized Labor's Incredible Shrinking Social Vision," in Morone and Jacobs, *Healthy, Wealthy, and Fair* 137–75.

8. "Ailing GM Looks to Scale Back Generous Health Benefits," *USA Today,* 24 June 2005.

9. Dana Vedder, letter to the editor, *The Mountain Times,* August 2006, 2.

10. John Maynard Keynes, *The Economic Consequences of the Peace* (New York: Harcourt, Brace and Howe, 1920), 226.

INDEX